New Developments in Medical Research

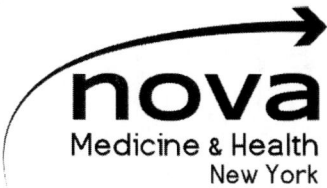

New Developments in Medical Research

A Literature Review on the Benefits of Propolis
Erik G. Martin (Editor)
2022. ISBN: 979-8-88697-253-5 (Softcover)
2022. ISBN: 979-8-88697-312-9 (eBook)

The Theoretical Foundation of Medicine
Thomas Nordström, PhD (Editor)
2022. ISBN: 979-8-88697-460-7 (Softcover)
2022. ISBN: 979-8-88697-482-9 (eBook)

Autoimmunity and Cancer
Soner Şahin, PhD (Editor)
Kenan Demir, MD (Editor)
2022. ISBN: 978-1-68507-937-6 (Hardcover)
2022. ISBN: 979-8-88697-077-7 (eBook)

Bioprinting the Human
Soner Şahin, PhD (Editor)
Kenan Demir, MD (Editor)
2022. ISBN: 978-1-68507-993-2 (Hardcover)
2022. ISBN: 979-8-88697-066-1 (eBook)

Botulinum Toxin: Therapeutic Uses, Procedures and Efficacy
James C. Lark (Editor)
2022. ISBN: 978-1-68507-817-1 (Hardcover)
2022. ISBN: 978-1-68507-826-3 (eBook)

More information about this series can be found at
https://novapublishers.com/product-category/series/new-developments-in-medical-research/

Denise J. Burton
Editor

The Dangers of Psychoactive Substances

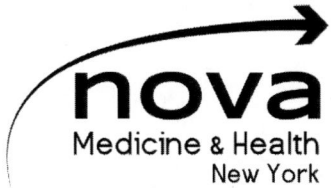

Medicine & Health
New York

Copyright © 2023 by Nova Science Publishers, Inc.

All rights reserved. No part of this book may be reproduced, stored in a retrieval system or transmitted in any form or by any means: electronic, electrostatic, magnetic, tape, mechanical photocopying, recording or otherwise without the written permission of the Publisher.

We have partnered with Copyright Clearance Center to make it easy for you to obtain permissions to reuse content from this publication. Simply navigate to this publication's page on Nova's website and locate the "Get Permission" button below the title description. This button is linked directly to the title's permission page on copyright.com. Alternatively, you can visit copyright.com and search by title, ISBN, or ISSN.

For further questions about using the service on copyright.com, please contact:
Copyright Clearance Center
Phone: +1-(978) 750-8400   Fax: +1-(978) 750-4470   E-mail: info@copyright.com.

NOTICE TO THE READER

The Publisher has taken reasonable care in the preparation of this book, but makes no expressed or implied warranty of any kind and assumes no responsibility for any errors or omissions. No liability is assumed for incidental or consequential damages in connection with or arising out of information contained in this book. The Publisher shall not be liable for any special, consequential, or exemplary damages resulting, in whole or in part, from the readers' use of, or reliance upon, this material. Any parts of this book based on government reports are so indicated and copyright is claimed for those parts to the extent applicable to compilations of such works.

Independent verification should be sought for any data, advice or recommendations contained in this book. In addition, no responsibility is assumed by the Publisher for any injury and/or damage to persons or property arising from any methods, products, instructions, ideas or otherwise contained in this publication.

This publication is designed to provide accurate and authoritative information with regard to the subject matter covered herein. It is sold with the clear understanding that the Publisher is not engaged in rendering legal or any other professional services. If legal or any other expert assistance is required, the services of a competent person should be sought. FROM A DECLARATION OF PARTICIPANTS JOINTLY ADOPTED BY A COMMITTEE OF THE AMERICAN BAR ASSOCIATION AND A COMMITTEE OF PUBLISHERS.

Additional color graphics may be available in the e-book version of this book.

Library of Congress Cataloging-in-Publication Data

ISBN: 979-8-88697-705-9

Published by Nova Science Publishers, Inc. † New York

Contents

Preface vii

Chapter 1   **The Synthetic Cannabinoids and Cathinones Phenomenon: From Hazardous Effects to Monitoring Approaches** 1
Merve Kuloglu Genc and Selda Mercan

Chapter 2   **A Comprehensive Method Validation of Caffeine as an Anthropogenic Marker in Water Samples by LC-MS/MS** 23
Yeliz Arpacik, Gulten Kahyaoglu Erbas, Tugba Tekin Bulbul, Merve Kuloglu Genc and Selda Mercan

Chapter 3   **A Cross-Sectional Chromatographic and Pharmacogenetic Study on the Functional Impact of CYP2D6 Variants and Their Expression Pattern** 43
Selda Mercan and Munevver Acikkol

Chapter 4   **Old Benzodiazepine, New NPS−Phenazepam: A Method Development Study** 59
Merve Kuloglu Genc and James Barker

Bibliography 81

Index 179

Preface

This book contains four selected chapters on the dangers of psychoactive substances. Chapter One reviews the synthetic cannabinoids and cathinones phenomenon from various angles. Chapter Two is a comprehensive methodical validation of caffeine as an anthropogenic marker in water samples. Chapter Three is a cross-sectional chromatographic and pharmacogenetic study on the functional impact of CYP2D6 variants and their expression pattern. Chapter Four is a method development study on old benzodiazepine and new NPS-phenazepam. The book concludes with a bibliography.

Chapter 1 - Substance addictions, which have origins in historical times to the present, directly affect the economy and security of countries as well as public health. Despite the recognized risks, over 275 million people have used drugs in the last year according to the United Nations Office on Drugs and Crime 2021 World Drug Report. While new dangerous substances have been appearing on the drug market, the international drug control system is struggling, for the first time, to keep up with the pace of the phenomenon known as new psychoactive substances (NPS). NPS have become a worldwide problem, with 136 nations and territories from every continent reporting at least one or more NPS, in total of 1,124 compounds have been reported around the world as of 2022. At large, NPS is an umbrella term for unregulated substances marketed as "legal highs" for alternatives to restricted or illegal psychoactive substances since the early 2000s. One of the most concerning elements of NPS is that consumers are unaware of the amount and dosage of the psychoactive chemicals found in marketed products. Formulation differences, toxic by-products inclusions, cross-contaminations may occur due to the manufacturing conditions of these substances in clandestine laboratories. For these reasons, in the literature, NPS have been associated to a variety of health problems, including non-fatal and fatal intoxications indicating that NPS can cause more dangerous harms than conventional illegal substances. The rising chemical variety of NPS, as well as their unprecedented number, makes monitoring and understanding this phenomenon even more challenging. These substances, which generally contain more than one synthetic substance together, are a global threat to public health and their continued alteration has posed challenges for analytical chemists, toxicologists and clinicians. Many substances with different chemical structures are classified under the definition of NPS. Synthetic cannabinoids and synthetic cathinones are the ones that most commonly seized and used among these substances. In this chapter of the book, the chemical structures, classifications, short/long-term effects and legal status of synthetic cannabinoids and cathinones will be provided. In addition, the conventional indicators and methods used around the world to monitor the consumption and trafficking of these substances will be discussed in detail, along with the limitations of these measures. Finally, innovative methods for monitoring the consumption of these substances, their current state of art and efficiency will be discussed as well.

Chapter 2 - Caffeine is one of the most widely consumed pharmaceuticals, which is also used as an anthropogenic marker in water samples. Therefore, developing a fast and reliable analytical method for detecting the pollutant effects of caffeine in any types of water is necessary and crucial. In this study, the authors aimed to develop and comprehensively validate a method conducted with the liquid chromatography-tandem mass spectrometry system. Validation parameters such as selectivity, analytical sensitivity, the limit of detection and quantification, linearity, precision, accuracy, and robustness were studied besides uncertainty. The correlation coefficient of the calibration curve was 0.997, while the limit of detection and limit of quantification levels were 0.165 and 0.548 ng/mL respectively. The repeatability studies were found below 10% RSD. The accuracy was between 87-109% on different days and at different concentrations ranging between 0.5 to 100 ng/mL. After the method validation, tap water samples (n=6) were enriched with concentrations of 50 ng/mL in 50 mL and the solid-phase extraction recovery rate was 93.3%. This is the first comprehensively developed and validated method published in our country to detect caffeine in water samples with high precision, accuracy, and recovery rates. The method can be easily applied to sediment, ground, or seawater samples besides tap water, surface water and wastewater.

Chapter 3 - Drug metabolizing enzyme polymorphisms result in slow or accelerated metabolization of the drugs. The authors aimed to determine CYP2D6*3 and *4 polymorphisms and copy numbers in psychiatric patients medicated by risperidone, olanzapine and sertraline, and quantitate the concentrations of these drugs. This study consisted of 77 psychiatric patients and 38 controls. CYP2D6*3 allele frequencies were identical for both groups (0.01); CYP2D6*4 allele frequencies were 0.15 for patients and 0.04 for the control group (p< 0.05). Twenty-one out of 77 patients had at least one mutant *4 allele. Gene copy numbers for Exon 9 between two groups were found statistically different (p< 0.05) (df = 102). Olanzapine concentrations in blood and urine of the patients carrying *4 allele were higher. Paliperidone/ Risperidone ratio was lower in blood and urine samples of the patients with *3 and *4 mutations, but higher in normal metabolizers. Differences between individuals and populations should be of concern for designing the most efficient treatment for psychiatric patients.

Chapter 4 - Designer benzodiazepines are a novel type of new psychoactive substance (NPS), often known as NPS-benzodiazepines. They are especially harmful, owing to inadequate toxicity information and a tendency to consider them as therapeutic drugs, which may result in misdiagnosis, treatment with consequent severe adverse effects and occasionally death. Phenazepam is a frequently abused, long-acting benzodiazepine, which has recently been categorized as a NPS-benzodiazepine. Phenazepam has been released into the recreational drug market from time to time for many years, but its reappearance as a NPS-benzodiazepine has demanded a cost-effective, easy and reliable analytical method for accurate identification and quantification of this substance for forensic and clinical purposes. This paper presents, a validated method specific to phenazepam using reverse-phase-high-performance-liquid chromatography coupled to ultraviolet - visible spectrophotometric detection. The proposed method analysed phenazepam within 2 minutes, accomplishing an overall 102.63 ± 0.06% accuracy, 0.220% intraday and 0.008% inter-day precision. The limit of detection and limit of quantitation values were determined as 0.158 and 0.526 µg/mL, respectively. The validated method was also successfully applied to a spiked hair sample. The validation performance of the developed method was satisfactory considering international council on harmonisation guidelines.

Chapter 1

The Synthetic Cannabinoids and Cathinones Phenomenon: From Hazardous Effects to Monitoring Approaches

Merve Kuloglu Genc, MSc
and Selda Mercan[*], PhD
Istanbul University-Cerrahpaşa, Institute of Forensic Sciences and Legal Medicine, Department of Science, Istanbul, Turkey

Abstract

Substance addictions, which have origins in historical times to the present, directly affect the economy and security of countries as well as public health. Despite the recognized risks, over 275 million people have used drugs in the last year according to the United Nations Office on Drugs and Crime 2021 World Drug Report. While new dangerous substances have been appearing on the drug market, the international drug control system is struggling, for the first time, to keep up with the pace of the phenomenon known as new psychoactive substances (NPS). NPS have become a worldwide problem, with 136 nations and territories from every continent reporting at least one or more NPS, in total of 1,124 compounds have been reported around the world as of 2022. At large, NPS is an umbrella term for unregulated substances marketed as "legal highs" for alternatives to restricted or illegal psychoactive substances since the early 2000s. One of the most concerning elements of NPS is that consumers are unaware of the amount and dosage of the

---

[*] Corresponding Author's Email: mercans@iuc.edu.tr.

In: The Dangers of Psychoactive Substances
Editor: Denise J. Burton
ISBN: 979-8-88697-705-9
© 2023 Nova Science Publishers, Inc.

psychoactive chemicals found in marketed products. Formulation differences, toxic by-products inclusions, cross-contaminations may occur due to the manufacturing conditions of these substances in clandestine laboratories. For these reasons, in the literature, NPS have been associated to a variety of health problems, including non-fatal and fatal intoxications indicating that NPS can cause more dangerous harms than conventional illegal substances. The rising chemical variety of NPS, as well as their unprecedented number, makes monitoring and understanding this phenomenon even more challenging. These substances, which generally contain more than one synthetic substance together, are a global threat to public health and their continued alteration has posed challenges for analytical chemists, toxicologists and clinicians. Many substances with different chemical structures are classified under the definition of NPS. Synthetic cannabinoids and synthetic cathinones are the ones that most commonly seized and used among these substances. In this chapter of the book, the chemical structures, classifications, short/long-term effects and legal status of synthetic cannabinoids and cathinones will be provided. In addition, the conventional indicators and methods used around the world to monitor the consumption and trafficking of these substances will be discussed in detail, along with the limitations of these measures. Finally, innovative methods for monitoring the consumption of these substances, their current state of art and efficiency will be discussed as well.

Keywords: NPS, synthetic cannabinoids, synthetic cathinones, illicit drugs, legal highs

> "Our very survival depends on our ability to stay awake,
> to adjust to new ideas, to remain vigilant and
> to face the challenge of change."
>
> – *Martin Luther King Jr.*

Introduction

Psychoactive substances have attracted the attention of all civilizations since the existence of humanity and have been used in many areas from rituals to medical purposes. From ancient times up until the 20th century, people discovered the psychoactive effects of some plants growing in the environment in which they lived and used them for different purposes due to their pleasant, sedative or stimulating effects. With the scientific developments in the 20th century, synthetic substances similar to natural psychoactive substances started to be produced for medical purposes. Hence, natural substances began to be replaced by synthetic ones due to the distinctive and potent effects they created on the central nervous system (CNS). Later, many of the synthetic psychoactive substances produced have been banned by laws with the discovery that they can do more harm than good in therapeutic use and have addictive characteristics as well as various severe side effects (Jickells Negrusz, Adam., 2008).

Since the 1900s, the use of psychoactive substances has become widespread and therefore gained a global dimension. For this reason, countries have decided to come together to combat the problem of substance abuse that affects them socio-economically. In the international arena, the Single Convention on Narcotic Drugs 1961 and Convention on Psychotropic Substances 1971 developed a global control system for psychoactive substances. The illicit substances marketed in those years were now called conventionals such as cannabis, amphetamine-type stimulants, cocaine, heroin, etc., which were included and banned in the aforementioned conventions. An emerging group of substances called *"new psychoactive substances (NPS)"* faced in the 21st century shows similar effects to these conventionals but were not listed among those banned at the meetings. The fact that these new substances are not under the control of the law in their time of appearance has caused the international control system to falter. Their chemical structure is often slightly altered by the addition or modification of a functional group of an existing regulated drug molecule. Simple alterations in their chemical structures distinguish these compounds from those in the legal system, allowing for their free manufacturing, sale, and use (UNODC 2020d; 2020c). Nevertheless, it is essential to note that the expression "new" does not necessarily relate to new innovations, as some of these chemicals were synthesized years ago, rather to substances that have recently introduced to the market and are being promoted as new emerging drugs. For example, John W. Huffman, a chemist, who unwittingly discover synthetic cannabinoids, while he was investigating the cannabinoid receptor in 1993. He synthesized JWH-018 (name after his initials), the very first NPS sold in the drug market called "spice" many years after its first being discovered (in 2008) (EMCDDA 2021a).

Although they can be classified according to their effects on the CNS, NPS are commonly categorized as synthetic cannabinoids, cathinones, phenethylamines, synthetic opioids, tryptamines, benzodiazepines, arylalkylamines, piperazines and other substances by the European

Monitoring Centre for Drugs and Drug Addiction (EMCDDA). Bright and appealing packaging has been used to market these products, which sold openly in head/smart shops and online, mostly aiming for recreational users. These novel compounds have been endorsed as "legal highs", "research chemicals", "designer drugs" to make them attractive and build an innocent image among users (UNODC 2021c; EMCDDA 2022b).

The rapid spread of many NPS on the international drug market pose a serious risk to public health and drug regulations worldwide. When it comes to the negative health effects and social harms of NPS, little is often known, which makes prevention and treatment extremely difficult. It is challenging to analyze and identify a significant number of chemically diverse substances available in drug markets all together. To respond to this unusual circumstance quickly, it is crucial to monitor, exchange information, provide early warning, and be aware of the risks. For all these reasons, the chemical properties, effects, legal status and monitoring approaches of synthetic cannabinoids and cathinones, which are the most common subgroups among NPS, are portrayed in this chapter of the book.

Synthetic Cannabinoids

Synthetic cannabinoids that act as agonists at the CB1 and CB2 receptors are also known as synthetic cannabinoid receptor agonists (SCRA). The effects on CB receptors are similarly to tetrahydrocannabinol (THC), the main psychoactive component of cannabis plant. However, cannabinoid receptor affinities and activities are higher than those of THC because they are the full agonist at CB receptors. Therefore, the frequency and severity of adverse effects are also higher than THC.

In 19th century, novel SCRA developed through research and/or pharmaceutical drives and patented by companies or scientist such as Pfizer (the CP- series of compounds), John W. Huffman (the JWH- series of compounds), Alexandros Makriyannis, University of Connecticut (the AM- series of compounds). It is the largest group of NPS currently being monitored by the EMCDDA. Since 2008, 224 new synthetic cannabinoids have been discovered in Europe, 15 of which were first discovered in 2021 (EMCDDA 2022a; 2021a).

Due to the nature of the cannabinoid receptors that allows binding of a variety of molecules, synthetic cannabinoids originate from chemically different classes of substances. In the past, naphthoylindoles, e.g., JWH-018, were the first synthetic cannabinoids to appear on the drug market, then it was followed by aminoalkylindoles (e.g., AM-2201), indole derivatives (e.g., 5F-MDMB-PICA) and their indazole analogues (e.g., 5F-MDMB-PINACA, AB-CHMINACA), then cumyl derivatives (e.g., CUMYL-4CN-BINACA) and recently 'oxizid' derivatives (e.g., BZO-HEXOXIZID) appeared and began to dominate the market. Because there are subgroups from so many different chemical structure origins, nomenclature of synthetic cannabinoids can also be quite confusing. Until recently, names for these substances may originate from the individual, institution or company names where they were first synthesized. However, recently, the *LinkedGroup-TailCoreLinker* system has started to be used by EMCDDA to achieve standardized nomenclature. To illustrate, Figure 1 shows chemical structure of BZO-HEXOXIZID by enlightening the new nomenclature for synthetic cannabinoids (EMCDDA 2022b; EMCDDA & EUROPOL 2019; EMCDDA 2021a).

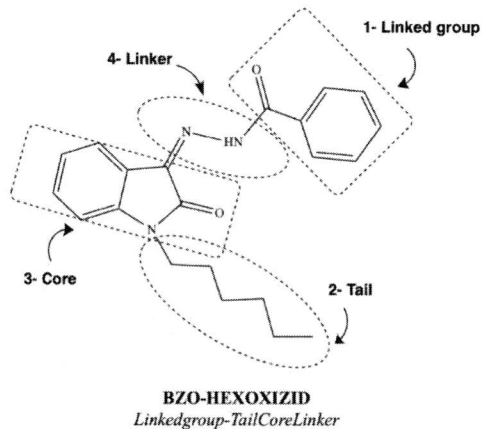

BZO-HEXOXIZID
Linkedgroup-TailCoreLinker

(Z)-N'-(1-**HEX**yl-2-**OX**oIndolin3-ylidene)**B**en**Z**O**h**ydra**ZID**e

Figure 1. BZO-HEXOXIZID structure to exemplify nomenclature of synthetic cannabinoids.

As other cannabinoids, synthetic cannabinoids also commonly abused by smoking, vaping, or boiling, rarely sold as powders or tablets. The use of electronic cigarettes to vape synthetic cannabinoids has also been reported to be on the rise in some regions of Europe. It is common to spray synthetic cannabinoids on plants (*Salvia officinalis, Turnera diffusa*) or tobacco to sell them as cannabis itself or as "legal" cannabis substitutes. Many NPS users consume the compounds unknowingly as adulterants of other drugs, which may cause catastrophic results (UNODC 2020b; 2022). If those who are unaware of the content of the substance they use are excluded, synthetic cannabinoids in general preferred by recreational users because these substances are cheaper than cannabis and have higher effects on CNS. Moreover, people who are subject to drug testing, such as prisoners or those receiving drug treatment, also prefers SC because some standard tests may miss newly introduced synthetic cannabinoids in the drug market. Consequently, many different methods have been tried to continue to use these substances. On the other hand, impregnating SCRA on paper, letter or clothes, is becoming an increasingly preferred method by inmates. Yet, this method can pose even serious health risk than normal since the amount of substance can change significantly across the paper, potentially causing lethal intoxications (EMCDDA 2021a).

Pharmacology and Toxicology

In its purest form, synthetic cannabinoids are typically described as crystalline powders that are white or yellowish and odorless. However, they are soluble in alcohols and organic solvents like methanol. The majority of synthetic cannabinoids are very lipophilic and typically insoluble in water.

Since the common route of administration is inhalation, the maximum concentrations (C_{max}) are typically reached a few minutes after the absorption through the pulmonary alveoli occurs. As opposed to inhalation, C_{max} takes longer to reach and typically happens in 30 minutes to several hours after oral administration as a rare route (Teske et al. 2010; Castaneto et al. 2015). Due to the rapid arrival of the C_{max} value in the blood, the time elapsed after consumption is very critical for clinical or forensic analysis in blood samples. In order to be able to determine the main substance or substances from the blood, it is necessary to take a sample pretty soon after consumption.

Depending on their structure, synthetic cannabinoids undergo various metabolization processes. Aromatic and alkyl structures are oxidized as part of the primary metabolic processes. Simple changes in the chemical structure of substances can cause different metabolization processes. For example, manufacturers frequently use the fluorine atom to replace the hydrogen atom as a way to avoid regulations while also increasing potency of the substance (Banister et al. 2015). This simple alteration creates different type of metabolites for two very similar compounds. This has made it extremely difficult for toxicologists and forensic chemists to maintain up-to-date, useful methods of analysis. The most important way to determine the consumption of the substance for clinical and forensic analyzes is to know the substance and its metabolites. If analysis is performed from a urine sample, the most typical phase II biotransformation of synthetic cannabinoids is glucuronidation. Cleaving glucuronic acid conjugates using glucuronidase is therefore crucial for analyzing samples of human urine. The majority of synthetic cannabinoids only go through renal excretion following a metabolic change. Forensic urine analysis requires the detection of metabolites in order to provide clear evidence of exposure. Nevertheless, the parent drug itself may occasionally be excreted in urine as well (EMCDDA 2021a).

These substances, which typically in combination of multiple synthetic cannabinoids, constitute a concern to public health on a global scale. Analytical chemists, toxicologists, and doctors have faced difficulties as a result of these substances' ongoing modification. NPS have different clinical and analytical detection issues than conventional illegal drugs. For instance, the rapid metabolization, lack of reference standards for analytical method development, and sharing common of metabolites (non-exclusive to substance) pose significant obstacles to the detection of these substances using various matrices.

Common reported effects on health are tachycardia, high blood pressure, convulsions, anxiety attacks, hallucinations and paranoia. The most important reason for synthetic cannabinoid intoxications and deaths is that more than one synthetic cannabinoid and adulterations can be found at the same time in a single product sold and there is no standardization in the production. This could partly be brought on by the uneven distribution of synthetic cannabinoids in herbal mixtures, increasing the risk of an overdose even in frequent users (Moosmann, Angerer, and Auwärter 2015). EMCDDA has received a rising number of reports indicating that cannabis products have been contaminated with extremely strong synthetic cannabinoids, namely MDMB-4en-PINACA since last year, which could also threaten a lot of life because many individuals from all ages uses cannabis products with various reasons often allowing them to be easily overdose by unknown synthetic cannabinoids found inside (EMCDDA 2021a; 2022a). One of the most often reported negative effects are cardiovascular effects, resulting with fatal intoxications as well. In fact, the cause or mechanism of death in situations utilizing synthetic cannabinoids is frequently stated to be cardiac arrhythmia and/or cardiac death (Paul et al. 2018; Ozturk, Yetkin, and Ozturk 2019). In 2020, three countries (Germany, Turkey and Hundarg) reported deaths to the EMCDDA linking synthetic cannabinoids in total of 93 cases (EMCDDA 2022a).

Synthetic Cathinones

The naturally occurring cathinone, the primary active component found in the khat plant's leaves (*Catha edulis*), is a derivative of synthetic cathinones. Chemically, synthetic cathinones are a β-keto analogue of amphetamine and therefore promoted as "legal" substitutes for amphetamine-type stimulants because of their CNS stimulating effects. As shown in Figure 2 and 3, these designer drugs share the same skeleton and all members distinguish by modifications of substitution sites (R^1, R^2, R^3, R^4, R^5) at cathinone backbone. It should be noted that synthetic cathinones, like other phenethylamines, have a chiral center, allowing them to exist in two stereoisomeric forms with different potencies and affinities (Soares et al. 2021; EMCDDA 2022c).

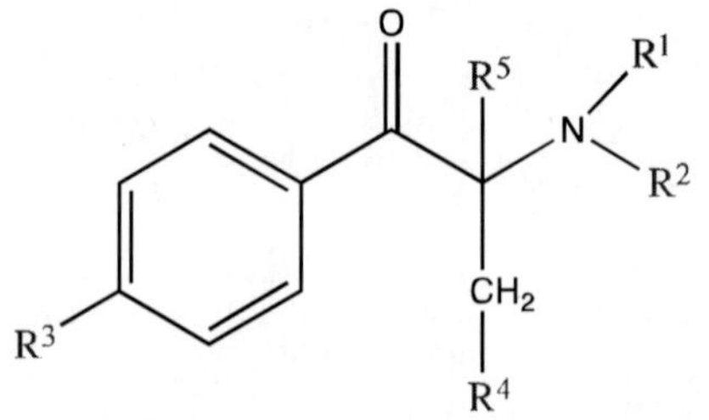

Figure 2. Cathinone derivative's general structure displaying patterns of substitution.

The first synthetic cathinone to be reported to the EMCDDA was methylone, an analogue of MDMA, in 2005. Then 4-methylmethcathinone (mephedrone) released, which was first synthesized in 1929, yet surfaced in 2007 to the drug market (Sur 1929; EMCDDA and Europol 2005). These drugs, which had previously been created for use in medical research but were shelved because their suitability for use in that context did not match the objectives, were made available for recreational use in the early 2000s. Hence, derivatives of ring-substituted cathinone that are not regulated have entered the recreational drug market in Europe. Their appeal can be attributed to their ease of accessibility and high purity compared to other illicit substances on the market. According to the latest EMCDDA report, synthetic cathinones rank as the second most monitored NPS group after synthetic cannabinoids, with more than half of the NPS seized in 2020 being the cathinone group (EMCDDA 2022a).

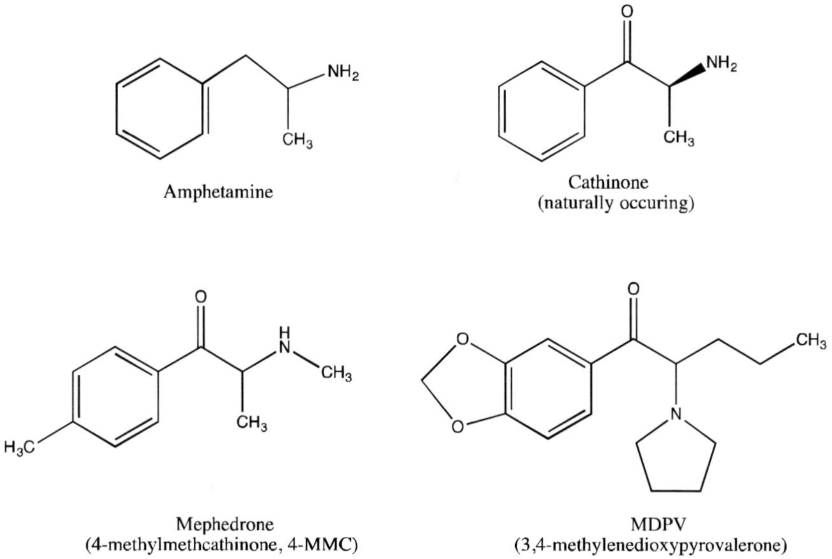

Figure 3. The structures of amphetamine, naturally occurring cathinone and its common synthetic derivatives (mephedrone and MDPV).

Pharmacology and Toxicology

These substances are purposefully mislabeled as "research chemicals" or "not for human consumption" and sold through Internet as "bath salts" or "plant food" to avoid legal controls. Manufacturers give substances attractive names and use eye-catching packages to increase sales of amorphous or crystalline powders that are white or brown colour. Capsule, pill, and powder forms are the ones that are most frequently sold. Thus, the most predominant pattern of use is usually oral administration, but rarely injection, rectal administration and mixing in a drink can also be other preferred routes. Another "popular" pattern among recreational users and club goers is so-called *bombing*, which indicates swallowing synthetic cathinone powder that has been wrapped in a cigarette paper as a method of ingestion (Prosser and Nelson 2012; Newcombe 2009). When compared to an oral intake, nasal insufflation is typically considered as a method that intended effects are achieved quickly and less doses are needed to reach those effects. Depending on the dosage and the substance administered, the metabolization may vary for the parent drug. In addition to dosage, administration method and interactions with other abused substances affect the absorption and, consequently, the bioavailability of synthetic cathinones. A few pharmacokinetic studies revealed the C_{max} value of mephedrone was approximately 1h following an oral administration of a single dose (Soares et al. 2021).

Changes in their chemical structure may generate different pharmacological properties in the body. For example, due to the ketone's polarity at beta position, blood-brain barrier permeability decreases. These derivatives are thought to be less potent than their corresponding phenylethylamine analogue. On the other hand, the amino group and pyrrolidine ring in MDPV may result in a more lipophilic compound, being more potent than many others (EMCDDA 2022c; Soares et al. 2021).

CNS stimulants, in this case synthetic cathinones, produce effects such as euphoria, improved sociability, self-confidence and sexual performance. On the other hand, reported adverse effects are agitation, severe psychosis, tachycardia, hypertension, mostly focusing on cardiac and neurological symptoms parallel to amphetamine-type stimulants. It has been reported that synthetic cathinones have caused fatal intoxications. The content and purity of marketed substances under the same name frequently vary noticeably, leading a tremendous public health problem across the globe (UNODC 2021a; 2021b).

Monitoring of NPS

Determining the level of drug consumption in a region is crucial for governments and legislators to implement drug policies based on objective, realistic and scientific data. In order to obtain these, many indicators have been monitored and recorded by relevant actors such as law enforcements, emergency clinicians, border units, etc. The first of these indicators, and the one that is frequently applied by almost every society, is the general population surveys (GPS). GPS help gather comprehensive information on drug patterns, prevalence and trends from people at different ages and socio-economic backgrounds. Then use these knowledges to prioritize concerns and prepare a plan of action on drug issue. GPS can reach many people at the same time and collect a significant amount of data from these people, and there are significant surveys conducted by important organizations to tackle drug abuse issue frequently. To exemplify, the European Web Survey on Drugs is one of the largest international web-based studies conducted by EMCDDA annually that collects information on individuals in many countries. Yet, as with any study, GPS also has limitations and disadvantages such as the long evaluation intervals, self-reporting bias and possible misinforming responses (fear of legal sanctions, etc.). Focusing on the limitations more specific to the NPS problem, creating standardized national questionnaires with local street names for NPS can be challenging since substance may be named differently in other communities. Additionally, users are unable to report their use of NPS in a survey since NPS are frequently employed as adulterants and users may not be aware that they are using NPS (EMCDDA 2022b).

Another frequently used indicator is the information about the substances and their quantities seized as a result of the operations of the law enforcement officers. This is the most important indicator that is followed both local and international levels to comprehend the drug trafficking routes for each drug worldwide. For example, every year United Nations Office on Drugs (UNODC) publishes a World Drug Report covering information specific to each illicit substance, notifying the certain routes from a starting point to the destination (UNODC 2022). For example, it is revealed that Covid-19 pandemic effected the supply-chain and production has shifted from China to India for synthetic cathinones, while synthetic cannabinoids are still originated from China mostly (EMCDDA 2022b). The region where the operation is carried out and the substances are seized may not always be the place where it will be consumed, meaning seizure data should be supported by other indicators such as emergency or mortality data to be able to confidently claim seized substances consumes in that area. In addition, not all trafficked substances can be caught is another limitation that should be considered.

Drug-related deaths and mortality are another indicator to tackle drug abuse problem collecting data on drug-induced deaths, which are fatalities directly caused by illegal drugs, and mortality rates among problematic drug users. However, the quality of this key indicator data is influenced by the reliability of its sources and the level of national health code standardization. Emergency hospital records are also important to assess the number of people who receive drug treatment. Since little is known about the daily or usual doses taken as well as side effects and toxicity of NPS it crucial to understand possible acute and chronic intoxication symptoms to be able to cope with their treatments.

With the effects of globalization and developing technology, there are also digital communications that can lead and contribute to these efforts for gathering accurate data. Analysis of the darknet and user forums can provide what GPS and other indicators cannot, the anonymity and fearless freedom of speech without any questionnaire boundaries be imposed to the user. Thus, one can learn the newly released NPS from the names entered into the search engines and can obtain the effects/symptoms of the substances on the market by utilizing the user forums. Hence, these sources can play a key role to foresee the drug trends and symptoms of certain substances (Al-Imam and Abdulmajeed 2017; Negri et al. 2021).

Wastewater-based epidemiology (WBE), which has featured since the early 2000s due to its advantages among other monitoring methods, is another complementary indicator for monitoring. WBE relies only on the excretion residues (metabolites) and parent drugs that can be detected in wastewater matrix by analytical techniques, therefore, its independent from all human aspects that can mislead the evaluation. With WBE, result evaluations can be completed rapidly, allowing for quicker implementation of necessary measures and the opportunity to track trends before they alter. When the risks and lack of information on doses, side effects and toxicity for NPS considered, the consumption of these chemicals in the community needs to be closely monitored by objective methods subs as WBE. Only WBE of all the indications cannot be used to identify a specific person, making the results anonymous. So, WBE is thus quickly developing into a key supportive indicator of illicit drug usage (Mercan et al. 2019; Asicioglu et al. 2021; Kuloglu Genc et al. 2021). Still, this approach as well has many limitations (Mercan, Kuloglu, and Asicioglu 2019). For example, WBE cannot distinguish the route of administration. Since sampling occurs from sewage samples of a certain population, targeted compounds will have low concentrations compare to biological samples. In the case of NPS, lower concentrations than conventional substances are expected causing analytical challenges for scientists. The need of stabile, exclusive biomarkers and reference standards (for novel NPS that is problematic) are limitations that are frequently encountered. Nevertheless, a non-profit organization called SCORE Network (https://score-network.eu/), supported by EMCDDA, coordinates standardized annual sampling periods with the participation of laboratories from different countries and cities. In addition, SCORE Network contributes to the production of accurate data by making interlaboratory comparisons each year. These efforts have included NPS on the radar of scientists dealing with WBE, and many studies have been conducted to determine their consumption in populations (Bade et al. 2021; Castiglioni et al. 2021; Bijlsma et al. 2021).

Apart from these monitoring methods, a *harm reduction* approach, which emphasizes the public health aspect of drug abuse phenomenon and focuses on reducing existing harm without the force of criminal sanctions, has begun to be adopted in some countries. Some of the models that take their place in this approach are drug-checking services and syringe collection campaigns of which also enlighten the changes in patterns of NPS use, potential emerging drugs in a certain population and the purity/adulteration/content analysis of injected drugs, while aiming to minimize mortality (EMCDDA 2021b).

Since none of these indicators and sources solely can fulfil the big picture, a worldwide holistic approach should be adopted. Acknowledging the complex nature of drug use, a multi-segmented perspective should be embraced to monitor, assess and evaluate the risks objectively. Therefore, in order to effectively address the drug problem, countries must exchange information among various governmental agencies and be able to act quickly to take required measures.

Legal Status and Early Warning System

As criminal law must be precise when defining an offense, the drug legislation typically entails a comprehensive list of all drugs name by name. In the 2000s, when NPS first began to appear, countries wanted to ban the harmful substance, they incorporated it into their local laws with their individual names as they did traditionally. However, the variety of these novel substances and the speed of their appearance challenged these conventional legal systems globally (EMCDDA 2016).

The endless cycle between NPS producers and legislators can be summarized as follows. First, different substances have been produced by differentiating them from the banned formula with minor changes in their chemical structures. After substance with minor alteration is released to the market, it is caught and analytically detected. Then a risk assessment is made and determined that it is another substance with a very similar chemical structure to the one within the scope of the law. Finally, this substance is also included in the law with its individual name. This cycle has begun to break by creative legal strategies that countries are generating. Considering how long it can take to update the law, countries such as Norway, Turkey, Lithuania and Croatia have decided to expand the scope of their current drug regulations by referencing defined groups describing specific substitution configurations as "generic name" rather than individual substance names. Thanks to the generic classification system, newly released NPS are included in the law before they are seen in the country. With the harms of NPS on the rise globally, many countries have enacted analog/generic laws or made additions to their existing laws or enacted laws specific to NPS. New legal strategies have been developed in reaction to the quick spread of NPS, and the situation is still changing depending on the market's dynamics (EMCDDA 2016; UNODC 2020a; 2021a).

The European Union (EU) is able to rapidly identify, evaluate, and address the public health and social dangers posed by NPS in Europe thanks to early warning system (EWS), risk analysis and preventative strategies. This EWS, which emerged in order to make countries aware of new NPS and to take legal steps quickly, allows them to include new appearing NPS in their laws long before they are seen in their countries. Through focal points of countries in collaboration with EMCDDA, the notification of a new NPS seizure data in a country is shared with other member states of the EWS, so that countries can take early measures against the substance before the harmful effects are seen. When the notifications related to the new substance exceed a certain level, the chemical properties of the questioned substance, street names, amount of seizures, route of administrations, production method and precursors, marketing strategies, health and social risks on users, the presence of poisoning and death cases are investigated by the scientific committee and a risk assessment report is published. If the conclusion reached as a result of the report is that the substance is threatening, the member states are required to include the substance within the scope of their laws within 180 days. This EU level exchange of information on the NPS issue helps countries stay ahead in the fight between illegal producers and the law (UNODC 2021a; EMCDDA 2022b; 2019).

EWS have been shown to be particularly useful in speeding up the exchange of information for creating novel analytical methods, observing their extent and hence prioritizing resources for control or scheduling activities.

Conclusion

NPS continue to provide many difficulties in terms of identifying, monitoring, and creating effective public health solutions. It takes close coordination, effective communication, and the new early warning system technology to mine, analyze, and model data for signals and trends in order to detect NPS forming on the black market. Even though the environment of illicit drugs and NPS is changing quickly, there have been achievements and lessons learnt globally.

Disclaimer

None

References

Al-Imam, Ahmed, and Ban A Abdulmajeed. 2017. "The NPS Phenomenon and the Deep Web: Internet Snapshots of the Darknet and Potentials of Data Mining Healthcare Discipline Projects View Project CME-CPD Activities View Project The NPS Phenomenon and the Deep Web: Internet Snapshots of the Darknet and Potentials of Data Mining." *Article in Global Journal of Health Science* 9 (11). https://doi.org/10.5539/gjhs.v9n11p86.

Asicioglu, F, M Kuloglu Genc, T Tekin Bulbul, M Yayla, SZ Simsek, C Adioren, and S Mercan. 2021. "Investigation of Temporal Illicit Drugs, Alcohol and Tobacco Trends in Istanbul City: Wastewater Analysis of 14 Treatment Plants." *Water Research* 190 (February): 116729. https://doi.org/10.1016/j.watres.2020.116729.

Bade, Richard, Jason M. White, Jingjing Chen, Jose Antonio Baz-Lomba, Frederic Been, Lubertus Bijlsma, Daniel A. Burgard, et al. 2021. "International Snapshot of New Psychoactive Substance Use: Case Study of Eight Countries over the 2019/2020 New Year Period." *Water Research* 193 (April): 116891. https://doi.org/10.1016/j.watres.2021.116891.

Banister, Samuel D., Jordyn Stuart, Richard C. Kevin, Amelia Edington, Mitchell Longworth, Shane M. Wilkinson, Corinne Beinat, et al. 2015. "Effects of Bioisosteric Fluorine in Synthetic Cannabinoid Designer Drugs JWH-018, AM-2201, UR-144, XLR-11, PB-22, 5F-PB-22, APICA, and STS-135." *ACS Chemical Neuroscience* 6 (8): 1445–58. https://doi.org/10.1021/ACSCHEMNEURO.5B00107/SUPPL_FILE/CN5B00107_SI_001.PDF.

Bijlsma, L., R. Bade, F. Been, A. Celma, and S. Castiglioni. 2021. "Perspectives and Challenges Associated with the Determination of New Psychoactive Substances in Urine and Wastewater – A Tutorial." *Analytica Chimica Acta* 1145 (February): 132–47. https://doi.org/10.1016/J.ACA.2020.08.058.

Castaneto, Marisol S., Ariane Wohlfarth, Nathalie A. Desrosiers, Rebecca L. Hartman, David A. Gorelick, and Marilyn A. Huestis. 2015. *"Synthetic Cannabinoids Pharmacokinetics and Detection Methods in Biological Matrices."* Https://Doi.Org/10.3109/03602532.2015.1029635 47 (2): 124–74. https://doi.org/10.3109/03602532.2015.1029635.

Castiglioni, Sara, Noelia Salgueiro-González, Lubertus Bijlsma, Alberto Celma, Emma Gracia-Lor, Mihail Simion Beldean-Galea, Tomáš Mackuľak, et al. 2021. "New Psychoactive Substances in Several European Populations Assessed by Wastewater-Based Epidemiology." *Water Research*, February, 116983. https://doi.org/10.1016/j.watres.2021.116983.

EMCDDA. 2016. *"Legal Approaches To Controlling New Psychoactive Substances." Perspectives on Drugs*, 4.

EMCDDA. 2019. "*Operating Guidelines for the European Union Early Warning System on New Psychoactive Substances.*"
EMCDDA. 2021a. "Synthetic Cannabinoids in Europe – a Review." *Technical Report.* https://doi.org/10.2810/4249.
EMCDDA. 2021b. "*Technical Report An Analysis of Drugs in Used Syringes from Sentinel European Cities Results from the ESCAPE Project, 2018 and 2019.*" Luxembourg. https://www.emcdda.europa.eu/system/files/publications/13571/ESCAPE_report_2018_2019-2.pdf.
EMCDDA. 2022a. "European Drug Report 2022: Trends and Developments." Luxembourg. https://doi.org/10.2810/715044.
EMCDDA. 2022b. "*New Psychoactive Substances: 25 Years of Early Warning and Response in Europe.*" Luxembourg.
EMCDDA. 2022c. "*Synthetic Cathinones Drug Profile.*" 2022. https://www.emcdda.europa.eu/publications/drug-profiles/synthetic-cathinones_en.
EMCDDA & EUROPOL. 2019. "*EU Drug Markets Report 2019.*" Luxembourg.
EMCDDA, and Europol. 2005. "*Europol–EMCDDA Joint Report on a New Psychoactive Substance: 4-Methylmethcathinone (Mephedrone).*"
Jickells, Negrusz, Adam, Sue. 2008. "*Clarke's Analytical Forensic Toxicology.*" London; Chicago: Pharmaceutical Press.
Kuloglu Genc, Merve, Selda Mercan, Murat, Yayla, Tugba Tekin, Bulbul, Cagdas, Adioren, Sumeyye Zulal, Simsek, and Faruk, Asicioglu. 2021. "Monitoring Geographical Differences in Illicit Drugs, Alcohol, and Tobacco Consumption via Wastewater-Based Epidemiology: Six Major Cities in Turkey." *Science of The Total Environment* 797 (November): 149156. https://doi.org/10.1016/J.SCITOTENV.2021.149156.
Mercan, Selda, Merve, Kuloglu, and Faruk, Asicioglu. 2019. "Monitoring of Illicit Drug Consumption via Wastewater: Development, Challenges and Future Aspects." *Current Opinion in Environmental Science & Health*, May. https://doi.org/10.1016/j.coesh.2019.05.002.
Mercan, Selda, Merve, Kuloglu, Tugba Tekin, Zeynep, Turkmen, Ahmet Ozgur, Dogru, Ayse, N. Safran, Munevver, Acikkol, and Faruk, Asicioglu. 2019. "Wastewater-Based Monitoring of Illicit Drug Consumption in Istanbul: Preliminary Results from Two Districts." *Science of the Total Environment* 656: 231–38. https://doi.org/10.1016/j.scitotenv.2018.11.345.
Moosmann, Bjoern, Verena, Angerer, and Volker, Auwärter. 2015. "Inhomogeneities in Herbal Mixtures: A Serious Risk for Consumers." *Forensic Toxicology* 33 (1): 54–60. https://doi.org/10.1007/S11419-014-0247-4/TABLES/3.
Negri, A., H. Townshend, T. McSweeney, O. Angelopoulou, H. Banayoti, M. Prilutskaya, O. Bowden-Jones, and O. Corazza. 2021. "Carfentanil on the Darknet: Potential Scam or Alarming Public Health Threat?" *International Journal of Drug Policy* 91 (May): 103118. https://doi.org/10.1016/J.DRUGPO.2021.103118.
Newcombe, Russell. 2009. "*The Use of Mephedrone (M-Cat, Meow) in Middlesbrough.*" www.lifeline.org.uk.

Ozturk, Hayriye Mihrimah, Ertan, Yetkin, and Selcuk, Ozturk. 2019. "Synthetic Cannabinoids and Cardiac Arrhythmia Risk: Review of the Literature." *Cardiovascular Toxicology* 19 (3): 191–97. https://doi.org/10.1007/S12012-019-09522-Z/TABLES/1.

Paul, Anthea B.Mahesan, Lary Simms, Saeideh Amini, and Abraham Ebenezer Paul. 2018. "Teens and Spice: A Review of Adolescent Fatalities Associated with Synthetic Cannabinoid Use." *Journal of Forensic Sciences* 63 (4): 1321–24. https://doi.org/10.1111/1556-4029.13704.

Prosser, Jane M., and Lewis S. Nelson. 2012. "The Toxicology of Bath Salts: A Review of Synthetic Cathinones." *Journal of Medical Toxicology* 8 (1): 33–42. https://doi.org/10.1007/S13181-011-0193-Z/TABLES/4.

Soares, Jorge, Vera, Marisa Costa, Maria De, Lourdes Bastos, Félix Carvalho, João, and Paulo Capela. 2021. "An Updated Review on Synthetic Cathinones." *Archives of Toxicology* 95: 2895–2940. https://doi.org/10.1007/s00204-021-03083-3.

Sur, Saem de Burnaga Sanchez J. 1929. "Un Homologue de l'ephedrine." *Bull Soc Chim Fr* 45: 284–86.

Teske, Jörg, Jens Peter Weller, Armin Fieguth, Thomas Rothämel, Yvonne Schulz, and Hans Dieter Tröger. 2010. "Sensitive and Rapid Quantification of the Cannabinoid Receptor Agonist Naphthalen-1-Yl-(1-Pentylindol-3-Yl)Methanone (JWH-018) in Human Serum by Liquid Chromatography–Tandem Mass Spectrometry." *Journal of Chromatography B* 878 (27): 2659–63. https://doi.org/10.1016/J.JCHROMB.2010.03.016.

UNODC. 2020a. "*Early Warning Advisory on New Psychoactive Substances.*" 2020. https://www.unodc.org/LSS/Home/NPS.

UNODC. 2020b. "*Global Synthetic Drugs Assessment 2020.*" Report. United Nations publication. https://www.unodc.org/unodc/en/scientists/2020-global-synthetic-drugs-assessment-regional-overviews.html.

UNODC. 2020c. "*Current NPS Threats.*" https://www.unodc.org/documents/scientific/Current_NPS_Threats_Vol.3.pdf.

UNODC. 2020d. "*Global Synthetic Drugs Assessment 2020.*" Vienna. https://www.unodc.org/documents/scientific/Global_Synthetic_Drugs_Assessment_2020.pdf.

UNODC. 2021a. "*Global Smart Update: Regional Diversity and the Impact of Scheduling on NPS Trends.*" https://www.unodc.org/documents/scientific/GlobalSMART_25_web.pdf.

UNODC. 2021b. "*World Drug Report 2021.*" https://www.unodc.org/res/wdr2021/field/WDR21_Booklet_1.pdf.

UNODC. 2021c. "*Current NPS Threats.*" Vienna. https://www.unodc.org/documents/scientific/NPS_threats-IV.pdf.

UNODC. 2022. "*World Drug Report 2022: Booklet 4.*" Vienna. https://www.unodc.org/res/wdr2022/MS/WDR22_Booklet_4.pdf.

Biographical Sketches

Merve Kuloglu Genc, MSc

Affiliation:
The International Association of Forensic Toxicologists
Turkish Society of Toxicology
Royal Society of Chemistry (2015-2017)
The Chartered Society of Forensic Sciences (2015-2017)

Education:
2016 – Present   PhD, Istanbul University-Cerrahpaşa, Institute of Forensic Sciences and Legal Medicine, Department of Science, Istanbul, Turkey
2014 – 2015   MSc, Kingston University London, Faculty of Science, Engineering and Computing, Forensic Analysis, London, United Kingdom
2009 – 2014   BSc, Bilkent University, Faculty of Science, Chemistry, Ankara, Turkey

Business Address: Institute of Forensic Sciences and Legal Medicine, Istanbul University-Cerrahpasa, 34500, Istanbul, Buyukcekmece, Turkey

Research and Professional Experience:
2018 – Present   Research Assistant. Istanbul University-Cerrahpaşa, Institute of Forensic Sciences and Legal Medicine, Department of Science, Istanbul, Turkey

Professional Appointments: Scholar of 2214-A - International Research Fellowship Program for PhD Students of TUBITAK.

Publications from the Last 3 Years:
1. Genc, M. K., Mercan, S., Yayla, M., Bulbul, T. T., Adioren, C., Simsek, S. Z., & Asicioglu, F. (2021). Monitoring geographical differences in illicit drugs, alcohol, and tobacco consumption via wastewater-based epidemiology: Six major cities in Turkey. *Science of the total environment*, 797, 149156.

2. Asicioglu, F., Genc, M. K., Bulbul, T. T., Yayla, M., Simsek, S. Z., Adioren, C., & Mercan, S. (2021). Investigation of temporal illicit drugs, alcohol and tobacco trends in Istanbul city: Wastewater analysis of 14 treatment plants. *Water Research*, *190*, 116729.
3. Kuloglu, M., Tekin, T., Turkmen, Z., Demircan, Y. T., & Mercan, S. (2020). Determination of doxylamine from a tea sample: A claim of drug facilitated crime. *Journal of Chemical Metrology*, 14(1), 68.
4. Mercan, S., Kuloglu M., Tekin T., Turkmen T., Dogru A. O., Safran A. N., Acikkol M., and Asicioglu F.. (2019). Wastewater-based monitoring of illicit drug consumption in Istanbul: Preliminary results from two districts. *Science of the Total Environment 656*, 231-238.
5. Mercan, S., Kuloglu, M., and Asicioglu, F. (2019). Monitoring of illicit drug consumption via wastewater: development, challenges, and future aspects. *Current Opinion in Environmental Science and Health*, *9*, 64-72.
6. Türkmen, Z., Kuloğlu, M., Tekin, T., Mercan, S., & Bavunoğlu, I. (2019). A GC-MS method for illegal stimulant drugs from serum: a multi-drug use sample in Turkey. *Journal of Chemical Metrology*, 13(2).
7. Okuroglu, E., Tekin, T., Kuloglu, M., Mercan, S., Bavunoglu, I., Acikkol, M., & Turkmen, Z. (2019). Investigation of caffeine concentrations in sport supplements and inconsistencies in product labelling. *Journal of Chemical Metrology*, 13(1), 28.

Selda Mercan (Assoc. Professor, PhD)

Affiliation: Department of Science, Institute of Forensic Sciences and Legal Medicine, Istanbul University-Cerrahpaşa, Istanbul, Turkey,

Education:
2007 – 2012   PhD, Istanbul University, Institute of Forensic Medicine, Department of Science, Turkey
2003 – 2006   Master's, Istanbul University, Institute of Forensic Medicine, Department of Science, Turkey
1999 – 2003   Bachelor, Istanbul University, Faculty of Science, Biology, Turkey

Business Address: Institute of Forensic Sciences and Legal Medicine, Istanbul University-Cerrahpasa, 34500, Istanbul, Buyukcekmece, Turkey

Research and Professional Experience: Health Sciences, Basic Sciences

Professional Appointments:

2022 –	Assoc. Prof., Istanbul University-Cerrahpaşa, Institute of Forensic Medicine and Forensic Sciences, Department of Science
2021 –	Assistant Director of the Institute Istanbul University-Cerrahpasa, Institute of Forensic Medicine and Forensic Sciences
2020 –	Assoc. Prof., Istanbul University-Cerrahpaşa, Institute of Forensic Medicine and Forensic Sciences, Department of Science
2018 – 2022	Dr. Lecturer, Istanbul University-Cerrahpaşa, Institute of Forensic Medicine and Forensic Sciences, Department of Science
2016 – 2018	Asst. Prof. Dr., Istanbul University, Institute of Forensic Medicine, Department of Science
2012 – 2016	Research Assistant Dr., Istanbul University, Institute of Forensic Medicine, Department of Science
2005 – 2012	Research Assistant, Istanbul University, Institute of Forensic Medicine, Department of Science

Honors:
- April 2014, Dr. Gökhan Eriş Scientific Encouragement Award, Forensic Medicine Foundation
- April 2006, Single Nucleotide Polymorphism of Cytochrome P450-2D6 (CYP450-2D6) *3, *4, *5 and *6 Alleles in Opiate Addicts, I.U. Rectorate Scientific Research Projects Unit, Scientist of the Year Award

Publications from the Last 3 Years:
1. Oruc, M., Mercan, S., Bakan, S., Kose, S., Ikitimur, B., Trabulus, S., & Altiparmak, M. R. (2022). Do trace elements play a role in coronary artery calcification in hemodialysis patients? *International Urology and Nephrology*, 1-10.
2. Mercan, S., Vehid, H., Semen, S., Celik, U., Yayla, M., & Engin, B. (2022). An ICP-MS Study for Quantitation of Nickel and Other Inorganic Elements in Urine Samples: Correlation of Patch Test Results with Lifestyle Habits. *Biological Trace Element Research*, 200(1), 49-58.

3. Genc, M. K., Mercan, S., Yayla, M., Bulbul, T. T., Adioren, C., Simsek, S. Z., & Asicioglu, F. (2021). Monitoring geographical differences in illicit drugs, alcohol, and tobacco consumption via wastewater-based epidemiology: Six major cities in Turkey. *Science of the total environment, 797*, 149156.
4. Asicioglu, F., Genc, M. K., Bulbul, T. T., Yayla, M., Simsek, S. Z., Adioren, C., & Mercan, S. (2021). Investigation of temporal illicit drugs, alcohol and tobacco trends in Istanbul city: Wastewater analysis of 14 treatment plants. *Water Research, 190*, 116729.
5. Mercan, S. (2020). A comprehensive artificial sweat study for quantitation of nickel and other inorganic elements released from imitation earrings purchased in Istanbul market. *Biological trace element research, 194*(1), 303-312.

Chapter 2

A Comprehensive Method Validation of Caffeine as an Anthropogenic Marker in Water Samples by LC-MS/MS

Yeliz Arpacik[1,2],
Gulten Kahyaoglu Erbas[2],
Tugba Tekin Bulbul[1],
Merve Kuloglu Genc[1]
and Selda Mercan[1,*]

[1]Istanbul University-Cerrahpaşa, Institute of Forensic Sciences and Legal Medicine, Department of Science, Istanbul, Turkey
[2]Department of Chemistry, Istanbul-1 Public Health Laboratory, Istanbul, Turkey

Abstract

Caffeine is one of the most widely consumed pharmaceuticals, which is also used as an anthropogenic marker in water samples. Therefore, developing a fast and reliable analytical method for detecting the pollutant effects of caffeine in any types of water is necessary and crucial. In this study, we aimed to develop and comprehensively validate a method conducted with the liquid chromatography-tandem mass spectrometry system. Validation parameters such as selectivity, analytical sensitivity, the limit of detection and quantification, linearity, precision, accuracy, and robustness were studied besides uncertainty. The correlation coefficient of the calibration curve was 0.997, while the limit of detection and limit of quantification levels were 0.165 and 0.548

---

[*] Corresponding Author's Email: mercans@iuc.edu.tr.

In: The Dangers of Psychoactive Substances
Editor: Denise J. Burton
ISBN: 979-8-88697-705-9
© 2023 Nova Science Publishers, Inc.

ng/mL respectively. The repeatability studies were found below 10% RSD. The accuracy was between 87-109% on different days and at different concentrations ranging between 0.5 to 100 ng/mL. After the method validation, tap water samples (n=6) were enriched with concentrations of 50 ng/mL in 50 mL and the solid-phase extraction recovery rate was 93.3%. This is the first comprehensively developed and validated method published in our country to detect caffeine in water samples with high precision, accuracy, and recovery rates. The method can be easily applied to sediment, ground, or seawater samples besides tap water, surface water and wastewater.

Keywords: anthropogenic marker, caffeine, LC-MS/MS, method validation, surface water

Introduction

Caffeine, also called 1,3,7-trimethylxanthine ($C_8H_{10}N_4O_2$), is a purine alkaloid that can be found in more than 60 plants. Beverages such as coffee drinks, energy drinks, tea, etc. contain caffeine, which is largely consumed as a pain killer, anti-inflammatory, diuretic, and flu drug. Caffeine is metabolized by the cytochrome P450 enzyme system in the liver into three main metabolites: paraxanthine (1,7-dimethylxanthine), theobromine (3,7-dimethylxanthine), and theophylline (1,3-dimethylxanthine), and is excreted via urine (Senta et al., 2015; Barone and Roberts, 1996; Heckman, Weil and De Meija, 2010; Mahoney et al., 2019).

The wastewater-based epidemiological approach (WBE), introduced by Daughton in 2001 and carried out for the first time by Zuccato et al. in 2005, is based on the analysis of exposed and consumed chemicals and their metabolites in wastewater (Daughton, 2001; Zuccato et al., 2005). The approach can be considered a large-scale urine test since the collected wastewater samples contain urine (Kasprzyk-Hordern et al., 2014). It has started as a tool to monitor community drug abuse and has been followed successfully in many countries such as Belgium, England, Spain, Norway, the United States, and Turkey (Mercan et al., 2019; Daglioglu, Guzel and Kilercioglu, 2019; Asicioglu et al., 2021). These studies were expanded to include significant geographic differences in drug use trends (Kuloglu Genc et al., 2021).

Caffeine and its metabolites in wastewater are analyzed using the WBE to generate real-time data. The evaluation of the population size and dynamics was also monitored through caffeine consumption of communities by related studies conducted in recent years by Senta et al. in 2015, Rico et al. in 2016 and Gracia-Lor et al. in 2017 (Senta et al., 2015; Rico, Andrés-Costa and Picó, 2017; Gracia-Lor et al., 2017).

When we look at the latest researches on pharmaceutically active compounds (PACs), pharmaceuticals and personal care products (PPCPs), and endocrine-disrupting chemicals (EDCs) in wastewater and their effects on the environment, we see that caffeine is the most commonly used pharmaceutical as a human biomarker (Daughton, 2001; Daughton, 2012; Gracia-Lor et al., 2017; Rodríguez-Gil et al., 2018; Guzel, Cevik and Daglioglu, 2019; Dafouz et al., 2018; Gao et al., 2016; Daughton and Ternes, 1999; Kurissery et al., 2012; Gheorghe et al., 2016; Valcárcel et al., 2011; Zhou et al., 2010).

Caffeine is evaluated as an ideal biomarker because of its stability, identifiability, ability to demonstrate human activities, and pharmacokinetic data variety (Gracia-Lor et al., 2017). In addition to being a biomarker in wastewater, another important thing about caffeine and its metabolites in surface waters or groundwater is that it is an anthropogenic marker. Surface waters can be contaminated by human activities and caffeine can be used as a possible chemical marker of sewage pollution. For example, Walter et al. reported that there was a parallel relationship between caffeine and *E. coli* in the waters of Bristol Harbor (Walter, 2017). In 1999, Daughton and Ternes stated that PPCPs should be considered hidden pollutants, not contaminants, and called them 'emerging pollutants' because of their continuous consumption (Ayman and Isık, 2015). If these pollutants are continuously discharged into the water ecosystem, they will pose an environmental risk (Kurissery et al., 2012).

There is a large number of studies investigating chemicals such as caffeine, cotinine, and drug residues in treatment plant effluent and surface waters and their toxic environmental risks (Rodríguez-Gil et al., 2018; Guzel, Cevik and Daglioglu, 2019; Dafouz et al., 2018, Kurissery et al., 2012, Ayman and Isik, 2015). Caffeine has been detected more in comparison to other chemicals in surface water or treatment plant effluent due to its high consumption amounts. According to a study in Spain, caffeine also exists in tap water (Valcárcel et al., 2011). Caffeine is also a pollutant for marine ecology and requires more research. The toxicity of the presence of these chemicals together in surface waters is much higher than their solo toxicity effects (Dafouz et al., 2018). The presence of caffeine and its metabolites in surface waters causes water contamination and affects living organisms.

Studies investigating caffeine and other biomarkers were initiated with the consideration of an environmental threat caused by pollutants (Rodríguez-Gil et al., 2018; Guzel, Cevik and Daglioglu, 2019; Kurissery et al., 2012; Ayman and Isik, 2015). This study aimed to develop and validate an analytical method with a low detection limit, high repeatability, wide linear range, high recovery, and short analysis time. A comprehensive validation study for caffeine in water sample conducted using the liquid chromatography-tandem mass spectrometry (LC-MS/MS) technique has not been previously published in our country. In this study, a method was established for the determination of caffeine, and its limit of detection (LOD), the limit of quantification (LOQ), correlation coefficient (r^2), relative standard deviation (RSD%), and recovery values were calculated. Selectivity/specificity, linearity, detection and quantitation limits, accuracy, precision, and robustness studies, which are extensive validation parameters, were calculated for the tap water samples as well.

Experiment

Chemicals and Equipment

Caffeine (CAF) was purchased from Sigma-Aldrich (St. Louis, MO, USA) in solid form. Isotopically labeled internal standard (ILIS) (cocaine-d3) was purchased from Lipomed (Arlesheim, Switzerland), gradient grade methanol (MeOH) for liquid chromatography from Sigma-Aldrich (≥99.9% purity; St. Louis, MO, USA), and ammonium acetate (AmOAc) eluent additive for UHPLC-MS and formic acid eluent additive for LC-MS from Fluka (Hannover, Germany). In addition, ISOLUTE C18 (500 mg, 6 mL) solid phase extraction (SPE) cartridges were purchased from Biotage (Uppsala, Sweden). For the SPE step of the samples, negative pressure vacuum manifolds with 24 ports obtained from Macherey-Nagel (Düren, Germany) were used. Evaporation under the nitrogen stream was conducted using a HyperVap HV-300 from Gyrozen (Daejeon, Republic of Korea) during sample preparation. The ultrapure water system was acquired from ELGA Purelab Flex (High Wycombe, the UK).

Instrumentation and Chromatographic Conditions

AB Sciex Triple Quad 5500 LC-MS/MS was used for the analyses (Ontario, Canada) along with the Spark LC system. Nitrogen was generated via a PEAK Scientific Genius 1051 device (Glasgow, Scotland); the instrument was calibrated and qualified before the analysis. The system was checked and the data were analyzed using the Analyst Software (Version 1.6.3). Previous publications have been scanned before generating the chromatographic conditions. Several trials were carried out with different ratios of solvents, flow rates, and temperatures to check the retention time (RT) and peak shape, and keep the analysis time short.

The chromatograms of caffeine and cocaine-d3 (ILIS) with good separation, selectivity, and sharpness were tried to be obtained in a short time by changing the flow rate and mobile phase ratios. Separation was performed using a Cortecs C18 column (2.7 µm, 100 × 2.1 mm) from Waters Corp. (Milford, MA, USA) with mobile phases (A) 2 mM ammonium formate in 0.1% formic acid in ultrapure water and mobile phases (B) 2 mM ammonium formate in 0.1% formic acid in MeOH. The total run time was 6 min, while the flow rate was 0.5 mL/min and the injection volume was set as 100 µL. The gradient of the mobile phase B was initiated at 5% and increased to 40% within 1.5 minutes and then continued to be increased to 95% within 2.5 minutes. Then, solvent B was decreased to 5% within 1 minute and held at that level for 1 minute for the equilibration of the column. The column temperature was set to 50°C. The chromatograms of caffeine and cocaine-d3 were obtained at 2.04 and 2.44 min, respectively.

Electrospray ionization (ESI) was applied in the positive-ion mode. The turbo ion spray source settings were: ion spray voltage (IS) 5500 V, source temperature (TEM) 450°C, curtain gas (CUR) 25, collision gas (CAD) 6, ion source gas 1 (GS1) 30, and ion source gas 2 (GS2) 35. Mass spectrometric analysis was done in the multiple reaction monitoring (MRM) mode under time-scheduled conditions, with a time window of 250 msec. The most abundant precursor/product ion transitions were obtained for each compound. The entrance potential (EP), collision cell exit potential (CXP), and declustering potential (DP) were 10.0, 8.0, and 80.0 respectively for all target compounds. The precursor and product ions selected for the analyte and IS along with their collision energies are listed in Table 1.

Table 1. Optimized MRM voltages, collision energies, and ions (m/z) of the targeted compounds

Compound Name	Precursor ion (m/z)	Product ion 1 (m/z)/ collision energy (eV)	Product ion 2 (m/z)/ collision energy (eV)
Caffeine	195.1	138/35	110/30
Cocaine-d3 (ILIS)	307	105/47	85.1/47

Stability of Analytes

The stability of caffeine was determined through laboratory studies performed at room temperatures, -4°C and -20°C. These caffeine standard solutions were studied on different days within a week. The results were evaluated using one-way ANOVA with a confidence interval of 95%.

Sample Preparation

The stock solution of caffeine was prepared at 100 mg/L in MeOH in solid form. The intermediate solution was prepared by diluting these stock solutions to 1 mg/L. Besides, the ILIS stock solution was prepared at 10 mg/L in MeOH and diluted to 1 mg/L. All the stock and intermediate solutions were stored at 4°C with paraffin coating during the study. The intermediate solutions were used to obtain mixed working solutions to achieve the calibration curves. The working solution range was between 0.1 ng/mL and 100 ng/mL caffeine, including the 10 ng/mL ILIS solution.

Solid-Phase Extraction (SPE)

Six tap water samples were used to check and approve the developed extraction method. Fifty mL water samples were spiked with a final concentration of 10 ng/mL ILIS and 50 ng/mL caffeine. Blank tap water samples including ILIS only were also used as blank samples to assess whether there was any contamination in tap water. No filtering process was needed before the extraction step. The SPE method was performed using ISOLUTE C18 cartridges (500 mg, 6 mL), which were conditioned with 2 mL of MeOH and 2 mL of distilled water. Following the sample loading step, the cartridges were washed using 3 mL of 5% MeOH (by gravity) and then centrifuged for 5 minutes at 5000 rpm for drying. The analytes were eluted using 2 mL of MeOH twice. The extracts were evaporated to dryness under nitrogen at 40°C and reconstituted to 1 mL with a mixture of the mobile phases A and B (1:1, v/v). Then, all samples were transferred to vials for LC-MS/MS analysis. All samples were analyzed as triplicates. The efficiency of the method was assessed with the recovery rate of the extraction.

Method Validation

The Fitness for Purpose of Analytical Methods, Validation of Analytical Procedures: Text and Methodology Q2 (R1), and Harmonized Guidelines for Single-Laboratory Validation of Methods of Analysis were checked for validation parameters (Eurachem, 2014; ICH, 2005; Thomson, Ellison and Wood, 2002). All results were also calculated using the national validation guidelines (Yılmaz, 2013; Acar and Diler, 2018).

The method was validated for selectivity/specificity, linearity, accuracy (trueness), precision (intra and inter-day), recovery, LOD, LOQ, and robustness comprehensively. After the determination of the validation performance, uncertainty was also calculated.

To evaluate the selectivity of the method, specificity was checked for any potential interferences by comparing the standard solution with caffeine as the standard solution and MeOH as the blank solution.

For the linearity studies of the method, eight different concentrations of caffeine standard solution ranging from 0.5 to 100 ng/mL in triplicate were prepared by diluting the stock and intermediate solutions. ILIS at 10 ng/mL and MeOH were added to all solutions to obtain 1 mL as the total volume. The calibration curve was constructed by plotting the peak areas against concentration. The linear regression equations and the correlation coefficient were calculated. The linearity of the calibration curve was also confirmed by the F-test.

Precision was determined by studying the repeatability (intra-day) and intermediate precision (inter-day) studies and was generated with 10 repetitions at three different concentration levels of caffeine standard: 0.5, 5, and 100 ng/mL.

Intra-day repeatability studies were carried out by the same analyst using three different concentrations of caffeine (0.5, 5, and 100 ng/mL) in the same laboratory and with the same equipment on the same day. The results were evaluated by calculating the RSD%. Grubbs' test was also used to detect the outliers in the study.

The caffeine standard solutions prepared by the same analyst at concentrations of 0.5, 5, and 100 ng/mL were analyzed on different days for intermediate precision (inter-day) studies. One way-ANOVA was applied for statistical evaluation to compare the results between days.

Accuracy (trueness) studies were performed through recovery studies at three different levels of standard stock solution added to the samples. The standard stock solution was spiked to determine recovery. CAF standard solutions prepared at concentrations of 0.5, 5, and 100 ng/mL were measured in 10 replicates on different days.

The LOD and LOQ were calculated based on the standard deviation (SD) of 10 repetitive caffeine standard solution measurements at the lowest concentration, using the following equations:

$$LOD = 3*SD \tag{1}$$

$$LOQ = 10*SD \tag{2}$$

According to the method validation and measurement uncertainty guide, these LOD and LOQ values were verified by the calculation using the standard deviation of the 3 repetitions blank solution study and the 3 repetitions LOQ concentration value study (Yılmaz, 2013; Acar and Diler, 2018).

The robustness of the method was determined by changing the column oven temperature from 50ºC to 40ºC and extracting the samples with two different analysts. The results were evaluated by the *Student's t*-test.

Recovery studies were carried out to check the extraction efficiency via caffeine spiking on six tap water samples. The details of the extraction process are presented in Section 2.7.

Even though it is not a validation parameter, uncertainty shows the distribution of the results using the method performance. The uncertainty value of the method was estimated through the determination of uncertainty sources. Precision, trueness, and linearity are the major uncertainty sources in a validation study. In the current study, relative standard uncertainties were determined based on the standard uncertainty of precision, trueness, and linearity parameters of the validation.

Statistical Analysis

Statistical analyses were achieved using Microsoft Office Excel 2016. *Student's* t-test was used to compare two groups, while one-way ANOVA was applied to compare more than two groups. For detecting the outliers, Grubbs' test was performed.

Results and Discussion

Method Validation

Method validation was performed after constituting the liquid chromatography conditions as mobile phases, flow rate, period of analysis, column temperature, etc., and mass spectrometry conditions as ionization mode, precursor/product ions of molecules, EP, CE, DP, CXP, etc., as described above.

Considering the specificity, the blank solution was compared with the caffeine standard solution prepared at 1 ng/mL concentration. The blank solution was performed, and no peak was observed during the analysis period. The chromatogram of the blank solution is shown in Figure 1. The chromatogram of caffeine confirms its presence in water at 2.05 minutes without any interference, as shown in Figure 2. The peak of cocaine-d3 was seen at 2.44 min, as shown in Figure 3. None of the analytes showed any interference; thus, the method was considered to be specific for all.

To check the linearity of the method, the calibration curves were plotted between the responses of peak area and eight different concentrations (0.5, 1, 2, 5, 10, 25, 50, and 100 ng/mL). It was measured with 3 repetitions. The correlation coefficient of the caffeine standard solution was 0.997. This indicates that the method had good linearity. The calibration curve was also accepted to be linear using the F-test.

Precision was determined by performing the repeatability (intra-day) and intermediate precision (inter-day) studies with 10 repetitions at 0.5, 5, and 100 ng/mL concentrations of caffeine standard solutions. The intra-day studies were carried out on the same day. RSD% values calculated for three concentrations were 5.52%, 7.47%, and 5.25% respectively. Grubbs' test was used to check out the outliers and detected no deviation in the data. For the intermediate precision studies, the caffeine standard solutions prepared by the same analyst were analyzed on three different days. One way-ANOVA was performed to compare the days for each concentration and returned *p* values of 0.172, 0.158, and 0.294 respectively. These results confirmed that there was no significant difference between the days.

The method was found to be highly precise and reproducible. All results also demonstrated that the studies were appropriate for method validation since RSD percentages were less than 20% and p values were higher than 0.05.

Accuracy studies were evaluated through recovery studies. The standard stock solution was spiked to determine the recovery rate at 0.5, 5, and 100 ng/mL concentrations. The studies were performed with 10 repetitions on three different days. The recovery results that ranged between 87.2% and 109% proved that the accuracy (trueness) of the method was provided for the method validation.

The results of the precision and accuracy studies are shown in Table 2.

Table 2. Results of precision and accuracy studies for three concentrations

Parameters	Conc.* (ng/mL)	Mean** (ng/mL)	RSD%	ANOVA F-value	Sig.***	Accuracy (%)
Intraday repeatability	0.5	0.545	5.52			
	5	4.421	7.47			
	100	93.30	5.25			
Interday repeatability	0.5	0.535	6.64	1.874	0.172	103.2-109
	5	4.469	7.33	1.971	0.158	87.22-92.52
	100	95.08	4.91	1.279	0.294	93.3-96.55

*concentrations
** mean of 10 different results on the same day for intraday repeatability; mean of 10 different results on three different days for inter-day repeatability.
*** significance.

0.3 ng/mL concentration of caffeine standard solution was spiked, and after the measurement of 10 replicates, the SD was calculated as 0.055. Three times the SD was calculated as 0.165 ng/mL as the LOD and ten times the SD was calculated as 0.548 ng/mL as the LOQ.

The verification of the LOD and LOQ was performed by analyzing 0.3 ng/mL and 0.5 ng/mL concentrations of caffeine with three repetitions. The LOD was verified since the maximum value of the three repetitive studies of the blank solution was less (0.108 ng/mL) than the mean of 0.300 ng/mL concentration of caffeine (0.379 ng/mL). The SD of the three measurements of 0.5 ng/mL concentration of caffeine was 0.026 and *s* (max. accepted SD of spike samples) was 0.067. These values showed that 0.5 ng/mL was the appropriate LOQ value for the developed method.

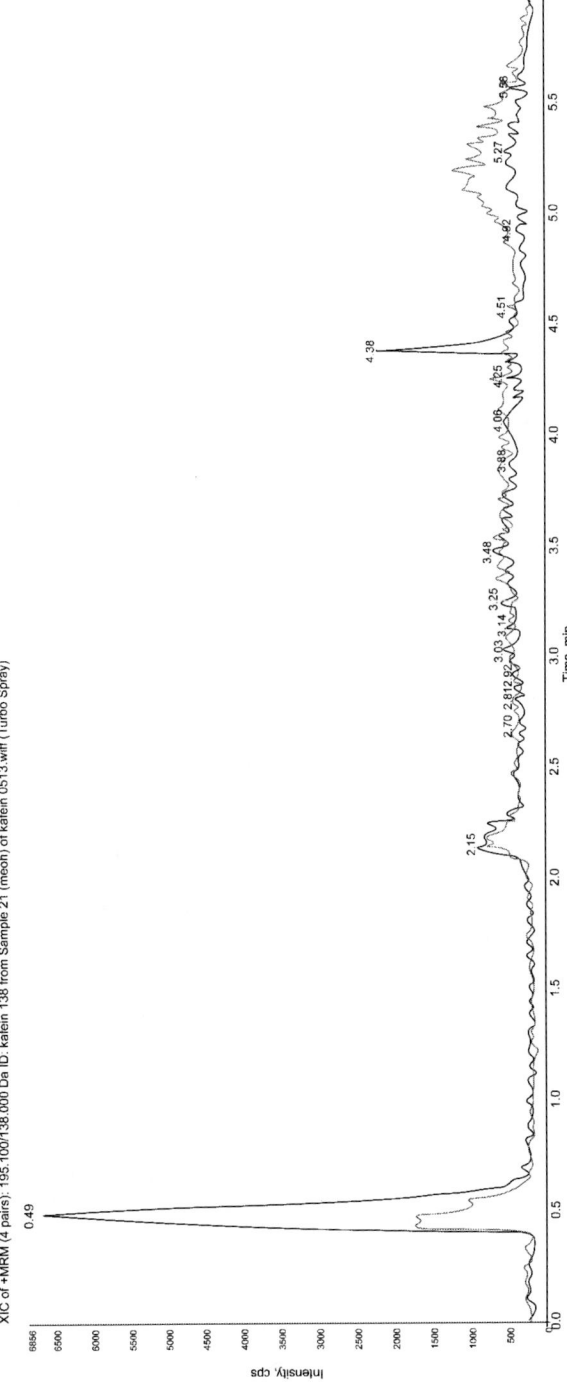

Figure 1. The chromatogram of a blank solution.

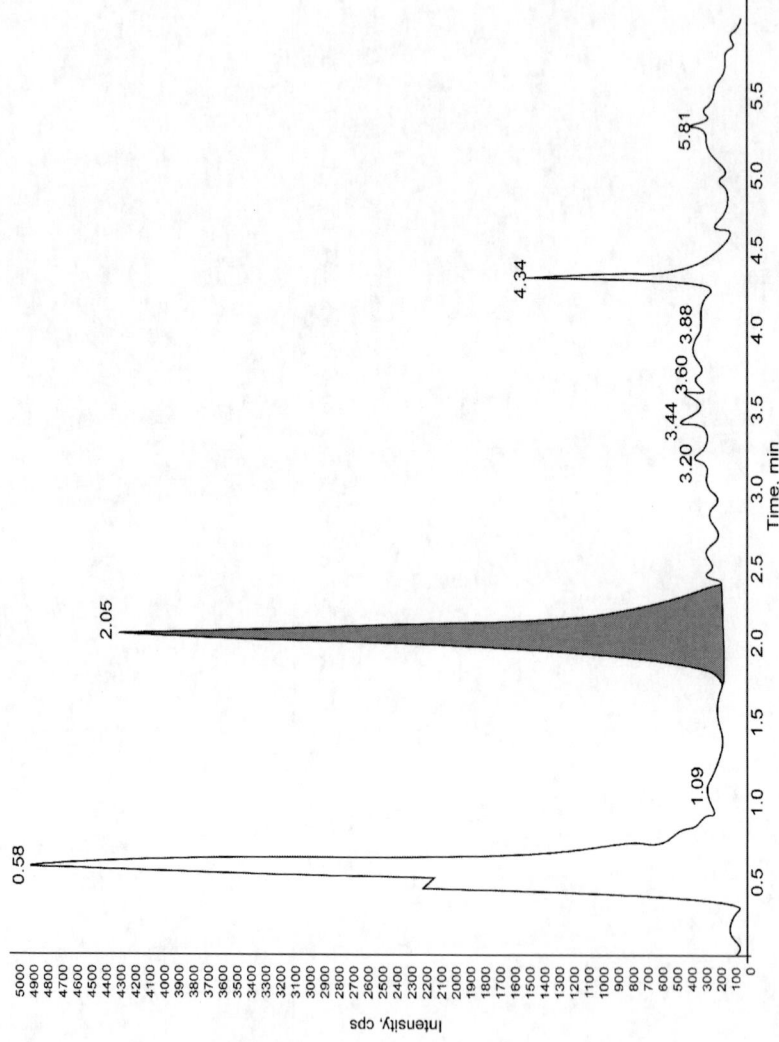

Figure 2. The chromatogram of caffeine in water.

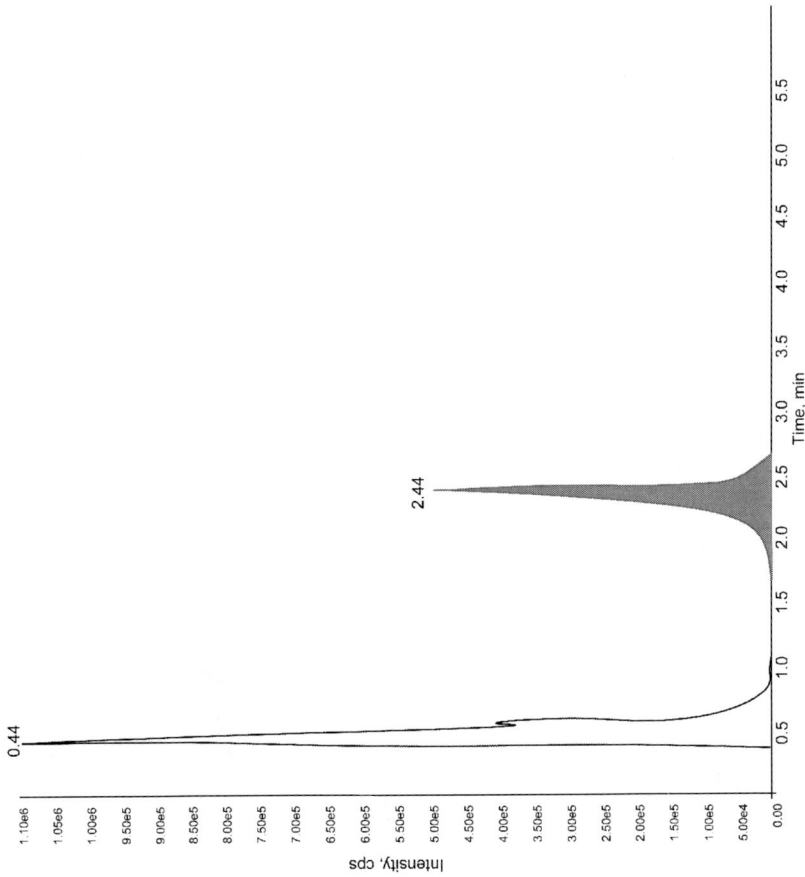

Figure 3. The chromatogram of cocaine-d3 (ILIS) in water.

The robustness of the method was determined by changing the column oven temperature and different analyst studies. The column oven temperature set up for the method was changed from 50°C to 40°C and 5 ng/mL concentration of caffeine was analyzed in three replicates. The mean results were 4.926 ng/mL at 50°C and 4.936 ng/mL at 40°C. Robustness was evaluated by the *Student's* t-test ($\alpha=0.05$) and accepted as appropriate ($t=0.075$ and t-$critical=2.78$). 5 ng/mL concentration of caffeine was also analyzed in six replicates by two analysts to determine its effects on the method. The mean results of Analyst-1 and Analyst-2 were 4.96 ng/mL and 4.88 ng/mL respectively for the 5 ng/mL concentration. The results were also evaluated by the *Student's* t-test ($\alpha=0.05$) and no significant difference was observed between the analysts ($t=0.809$ and t-$critical=2.23$).

Measurement Uncertainty

Unlike other validation studies, measurement uncertainty was also calculated in this study. RSDpool (a single RSD value obtained from intra-day repeatability) was calculated as 0.062 for standard uncertainty (u) of precision. RSDwrpool (a single RSD value obtained from inter-day repeatability) was also calculated as 0.063 for standard uncertainty (u) of precision. u_i (standard uncertainty of trueness) was calculated using the averages of recovery percentage, SD, the total number of measurements, RSD, etc. u (x_0) (standard uncertainty of linearity) was calculated using the concentration (x) and response (y) values. x_0 (any concentration level at the calibration level range) was chosen as 25 ng/mL.

All relative uncertainties were combined for combined relative uncertainty and expanded relative uncertainty, and are represented in Table 3.

Table 3. Sources of uncertainties, combined and expanded relative uncertainty

	x value	standard uncertainty (u)	relative uncertainties
Precision (Inter-day repeatability)	1	0.063	0.063
Precision (Intra-day repeatability)	1	0.062	0.062
Trueness	97.16	1.007	0.0103
Linearity	25	1.505	0.06
Combined relative uncertainty			*0.107*
Expanded relative uncertainty			0.21

Stability

To check the stability, 10 ng/mL concentration of caffeine standard solution was checked at room temperature, -4°C, and -20°C. The solutions were analyzed with three replicates on different days in a week. The results were evaluated by ANOVA. No significant statistical difference was found since the p value was higher than 0.05 (p=0.06) and caffeine solutions were accepted as stable during the study.

Extraction Efficiency

To evaluate the extraction efficiency of the recovery studies, the extracted samples (50 ng/mL caffeine), as described in the method validation section, were measured in six replicates using the developed method. The average extraction recovery rate was 93.3%, suggesting that the recovery of this developed method was satisfactorily high.

Benchmarking Studies

The literature holds numerous studies performed to determine the caffeine level in several water samples such as sewage, surface water, groundwater, seawater, hospital wastewater, and influents and effluents of drinking water treatment plants (Senta et al., 2015; Rico, Andrés-Costa and Picó, 2017; Guzel, Cevik and Daglioglu, 2019; Zhou et al., 2010; Ayman and Isik, 2015; Goren and Daglıoglu, 2019). The comparison of some method parameters is listed in Table 4. According to the results, our fully validated method and other studies have similar r^2 values for linearity. When the linear ranges are considered, it is seen that the lowest limit is quite low. Since the matrices of other studies are wastewater, food, etc., the concentration of caffeine is expected to be higher than surface water, therefore, the working ranges of other studies are higher than the presented study. Additionally, all performance parameters were found satisfactory with a low uncertainty value in this comprehensively validated method. Studies on the caffeine concentrations in surface water showed that the highest caffeine concentration encountered in seawater was 11 ng/mL in Australia and 8.23 ng/mL in Japan, while the highest estuary water concentration was measured as 5.86 ng/mL in the USA (Dafouz et al., 2018). In Europe, The Aegean Sea/Dardanelles has the highest caffeine concentration with 3.068 ng/mL. Also, in Italy and Spain, 1.11 and 0.857 ng/mL caffeine concentrations were found in seawater, respectively (Dafouz et al., 2018). Therefore, the obtained linear range in our study may be accepted to represent all these concentrations determined in surface water. Our study has high precision with an RSD of 6.3% and high accuracy ranging between 87.2% and 109%. Since caffeine concentration in blank samples was about 0.08 ng/mL, the LOD and LOQ values are acceptable and proper to determine the caffeine levels in several matrices.

Table 4. Comparison of the validation parameters of our method with the caffeine-detecting method in various samples

Studies	LOD (ng/mL)	LOQ (ng/mL)	Range (ng/mL)	RSD%	r^2	Accuracy %	Recovery %
Goren and Daglioglu, 2019	1.6	2.5			0.990	89-116	92
Senta et al. 2015		0.0036 (MQL)	0-600	12	>0.998		88
Rico, Andrés-Costa and Picó, 2017	0.022	0.073	2-2000	4.1-5.9	>0.999		38
Ayman and Isık, 2015	0.183	0.61	1-500		>0.997		
Guzel, Cevik and Daglioglu, 2019	0.2	0.6	0.01-100		>0.990	70-110	
Zhou et al., 2010		0.029	2-1000	9	>0.990		84.1±7.6
This study	0.165	0.548	0.5-100	<10	>0.997	87.2-109	93.3

Conclusion

Caffeine is as important as other human biomarkers since it provides information about the population of a region from wastewater and is an anthropogenic marker in surface water. With the consideration of generating an environmental risk, the presence of caffeine in waters has been studied in many countries including Turkey (Rodríguez-Gil et al., 2018; Guzel, Cevik and Daglioglu, 2019; Kurissery et al., 2012; Ayman and Isik, 2015). In this study, we successfully achieved quick, easy, and specific method parameters with a low LOQ, high repeatability, and high recovery method for water samples using LC-MS/MS. In all studies, we used 10 ng/mL of cocaine-d3 as the internal standard to eliminate bias caused by sample injection and extraction to standardize the changes in the MS/MS conditions and aimed to obtain results with high repeatability. Methanol (non-CAF solvent) and caffeine standard solutions at 1 ng/mL concentrations were analyzed for the selectivity parameter of method validation and concluded that the method was specific and sensitive for caffeine detection in surface water. This is the most comprehensive validated method for caffeine monitoring in water samples. Thanks to the satisfactory results from the current study, environmental pollution by caffeine in surface water can be detected and the environmental risk can be determined. Also, the same method can be applied to wastewater, with an approved extraction process with a very low uncertainty value, as well as surface water, sediment, ground, or seawater. Thus, real information about population size and dynamics can be obtained from caffeine and its metabolites in wastewater considering the importance of the WBE approach and the *de facto* population in drug studies. Therefore, this newly developed and fully validated method can be enhanced with other caffeine metabolites to monitor caffeine consumption, especially with 1,7-dimethyluric acid, which has been found to be a more stable caffeine metabolite in previous studies.

Acknowledgments

The study was supported by Istanbul University-Cerrahpaşa, Scientific Research Foundation with the project number: FYL-2018-32800. The authors are grateful to the administration of Istanbul-1 Public Health Laboratory and especially thankful to the Department of Chemistry analysts for their kind support.

References

Acar CO, Diler F. Pestisit analizleri için metot validasyonu ve ölçüm belirsizliği hesaplanması açıklamalı uygulama rehberi [*Explanatory guide to method validation and measurement uncertainty calculation for pesticide analysis*]. (2018) 4th revision. Accessed June 05, 2020. https://gidalab.tarimorman.gov.tr/gidareferans/Menu/76/Pestisit.

Asicioglu, F, Genc, M. K., Bulbul, T. T., Yayla, M., Simsek, S. Z., Adioren, C., & Mercan, S. Investigation of temporal illicit drugs, alcohol and tobacco trends in Istanbul city: Wastewater analysis of 14 treatment plants. *Water Research* (2021) 190 :116729.

Ayman Z, Isik M. Pharmaceutically active compounds in water, Aksaray, Turkey. *CLEAN–Soil, Air, Water* (2015) 43(10):1381-1388.

Barone JJ, Roberts HR. Caffeine consumption. *Food and chemical toxicology* (1996) 34(1):119-129.

Dafouz, R, Cáceres, N, Rodríguez-Gil, JL, Mastroianni, N, López de Alda, M, Barceló, D, de Miguel, ÁG, & Valcárcel, Y. Does the presence of caffeine in the marine environment represent an environmental risk? A regional and global study. *Science of the total environment* (2018) 615:632-642.

Daglioglu N, Guzel EY, Kilercioglu S. Assessment of illicit drugs in wastewater and estimation of drugs of abuse in Adana Province, Turkey. *Forensic science international* (2019) 294: 132-139.

Daughton CG, Thomas AT. Pharmaceuticals and personal care products in the environment: agents of subtle change? *Environmental health perspectives* (1999) 107 (suppl 6): 907-938.

Daughton CG. Illicit drugs in municipal sewage. *Pharmaceuticals and Care Products in the Environment* (2001) 791: 348-364.

Daughton CG. Real-time estimation of small-area populations with human biomarkers in sewage. *Science of the Total Environment* (2012) 414: 6-21.

Emma Gracia-Lor, Nikolaos I Rousis, Ettore Zuccato, Richard Bade, Jose Antonio Baz-Lomba, Erika Castrignanò, Ana Causanilles, Félix Hernández, Barbara Kasprzyk-Hordern, Juliet Kinyua, Ann-Kathrin McCall, Alexander LN van Nuijs, Benedek G Plósz, Pedram Ramin, Yeonsuk Ryu, Miguel M Santos, Kevin Thomas, Pimde Voogt, Zhugen Yang, Sara Castiglioni. Estimation of caffeine intake from analysis of caffeine metabolites in wastewater. *Science of the Total Environment* (2017) 609:1582-1588.

Gao, J, O'Brien, J, Du, P, Li, X, Ort, C, Mueller, JF, & Thai, PK. Measuring selected PPCPs in wastewater to estimate the population in different cities in China. *Science of the Total Environment* (2016) 568:164-170.

Genc, M. K., Mercan, S., Yayla, M., Bulbul, T. T., Adioren, C., Simsek, S. Z., & Asicioglu, F. Monitoring geographical differences in illicit drugs, alcohol, and tobacco consumption via wastewater-based epidemiology: Six major cities in Turkey. *Science of the total environment* (2021) 797:149156.

Gheorghe, S, Petre, J, Lucaciu, I, Stoica, C, & Nita-Lazar, M. Risk screening of pharmaceutical compounds in Romanian aquatic environment. *Environmental monitoring and assessment* (2016) 188(6):1-16.

Goren IE, Daglıoglu N. Enerji İçeceklerinde Yüksek Risk: Kafein [High Risk in Energy Drinks: Caffeine]. *Türkiye Klinikleri Adli Tıp ve Adli Bilimler Dergisi* (2019) 16(2):98-103.

Gracia-Lor, E, Castiglioni, S, Bade, R, Been, F, Castrignanò, E, Covaci, A, González-Mariño, I, Hapeshi, E, Kasprzyk-Hordern, B, Kinyua, J, Lai, FY, Letzel, T, Lopardo, L, Meyer, MR, O'Brien, J, Ramin, P, Rousis, NI, Rydevik, A, Ryu, Y, Bijlsma, L. Measuring biomarkers in wastewater as a new source of epidemiological information: Current state and future perspectives. *Environment international* (2017) 99:131-150.

Guideline, Eurachem. *The Fitness for Purpose of Analytical Methods: A Laboratory Guide to Method Validation and Related Topics.* (2014) Second edition.

Guideline, ICH Harmonised Tripartite. *Validation of analytical procedures: text and methodology.* Q2 (R1) (2005) Step 4 version.

Guzel EY, Cevik F, Daglioglu N. Determination of pharmaceutical active compounds in Ceyhan River, Turkey: Seasonal, spatial variations and environmental risk assessment. *Human and Ecological Risk Assessment: An International Journal* (2019) 25(8):1980-1995.

Heckman MA, Weil J, De Mejia EG. Caffeine (1, 3, 7-trimethylxanthine) in foods: a comprehensive review on consumption, functionality, safety, and regulatory matters. *Journal of food science* (2010) 75(3):R77-R87.

Kasprzyk-Hordern, B, Bijlsma, L, Castiglioni, S, Covaci, A, de Voogt, P, Emke, E, Hernandez, F, Ort, C, Reid, M, van Nuijs, A, and Thomas, KV. Wastewater-based epidemiology for public health monitoring. *Water and Sewerage Journal* (2014) 4:25-26.

Kurissery S, Kanavillil N, Verenitch S, Mazumder, A. Caffeine as an anthropogenic marker of domestic waste: A study from Lake Simcoe watershed. *Ecological Indicators* (2012) 23:501-508.

Mahoney, Caroline R, Grace E Giles, Bernadette P Marriott, Daniel A Judelson, Ellen L Glickman, Paula J Geiselman, Harris R Lieberman. Intake of caffeine from all sources and reasons for use by college students. *Clinical nutrition* (2019) 38(2):668-675.

Mercan, Selda, Merve Kuloglu, Tugba Tekin, Zeynep Turkmen, Ahmet Ozgur Dogru, Ayse N Safran, Munevver Acikkol, Faruk Asicioglu. Wastewater-based monitoring of illicit drug consumption in Istanbul: Preliminary results from two districts. *Science of the Total Environment* (2019) 656:231-238.

Rico M, Andrés-Costa MJ, Picó Y. Estimating population size in wastewater-based epidemiology. Valencia metropolitan area as a case study. *Journal of hazardous materials* (2017) 323:156-165.

Rodríguez-Gil, JL, N Cáceres, R Dafouz, Y Valcárcel. Caffeine and paraxanthine in aquatic systems: Global exposure distributions and probabilistic risk assessment. *Science of the total environment* (2018) 612:1058-1071.

Senta, Ivan, Emma Gracia-Lor, Andrea Borsotti, Ettore Zuccato, Sara Castiglioni. Wastewater analysis to monitor use of caffeine and nicotine and evaluation of their metabolites as biomarkers for population size assessment. *Water research* (2015) 74:23-33.

Thompson M, Ellison SL, Wood R. Harmonized guidelines for single-laboratory validation of methods of analysis (IUPAC Technical Report). *Pure and applied chemistry* (2002) 74:835-855.

Valcárcel, Y, S González Alonso, JL Rodríguez-Gil, A Gil, M Catalá. Detection of pharmaceutically active compounds in the rivers and tap water of the Madrid Region (Spain) and potential ecotoxicological risk. *Chemosphere* (2011) 84(10):1336-1348.

Walter Y, Bowdler P, and Honeychurch KC. Determination of caffeine and paracetamol in Bristol harbour water by LC/MS/MS. (2017) *Paper presented at RSC Twitter Conference*, Bristol, UK, March 20-21.

Yılmaz, A. Kimyasal analizlerde metod validasyonu ve verifikasyonu [Method validation and verification in chemical analysis]. *Turklab Rehber 01* (2012). Accessed June 05, 2020. http://turklab.org/tr/TURKLAB_Rehber_01_Rev.2.pdf.

Zhou, Haidong, Chunying Wu, Xia Huang, Mijun Gao, Xianghua Wen, Hiroshi Tsuno, Hiroaki Tanaka. Occurrence of selected pharmaceuticals and caffeine in sewage treatment plants and receiving rivers in Beijing, China. *Water Environment Research* (2010) 82(11):2239-2248.

Zuccato, Ettore, Chiara Chiabrando, Sara Castiglioni, Davide Calamari, Renzo Bagnati, Silvia Schiarea and Roberto Fanelli. Cocaine in surface waters: a new evidence-based tool to monitor community drug abuse. *Environmental Health* (2005) 4(1):1-7.

Chapter 3

A Cross-Sectional Chromatographic and Pharmacogenetic Study on the Functional Impact of CYP2D6 Variants and Their Expression Pattern

Selda Mercan[*], PhD
and Munevver Acikkol, PhD (TR)

Istanbul University – Cerrahpaşa, Institute of Forensic Sciences and Legal Medicine
Istanbul, Buyukcekmece, Turkey

Abstract

Drug metabolizing enzyme polymorphisms result in slow or accelerated metabolization of the drugs. We aimed to determine CYP2D6*3 and *4 polymorphisms and copy numbers in psychiatric patients medicated by risperidone, olanzapine and sertraline, and quantitate the concentrations of these drugs. This study consisted of 77 psychiatric patients and 38 controls. CYP2D6*3 allele frequencies were identical for both groups (0.01); CYP2D6*4 allele frequencies were 0.15 for patients and 0.04 for the control group ($p < 0.05$). Twenty-one out of 77 patients had at least one mutant *4 allele. Gene copy numbers for Exon 9 between two groups were found statistically different ($p < 0.05$) (df = 102). Olanzapine concentrations in blood and urine of the patients carrying *4 allele were higher. Paliperidone/Risperidone ratio was lower in blood and urine samples of the patients with *3 and *4 mutations, but higher in normal metabolizers. Differences between individuals and populations should be

---

[*] Corresponding Author's Email: mercans@iuc.edu.tr.

In: The Dangers of Psychoactive Substances
Editor: Denise J. Burton
ISBN: 979-8-88697-705-9
© 2023 Nova Science Publishers, Inc.

of concern for designing the most efficient treatment for psychiatric patients.

Keywords: CYP2D6, gene copy number, psychiatric patients, drug/metabolite ratio

Introduction

The pharmacodynamics of the substances used in the treatment of various conditions might have various effects on the organism. These variations are influenced by dose, age, gender, pathological and environmental conditions, and genetic diversity among the individuals and populations (Lin, 2007). Since it is not possible to eliminate the intra-individual variables, personalized treatment options based on the genetic polymorphisms of the individual were developed in order to obtain the best treatment approach for a specific patient (Butler, 2018). Despite the increasing number of drug options in the field of psychiatry, a desirable success in the treatment might not be achieved in a variety of patients. Although the guideline-based drug regimen recommendations are given in the determined dose and durations, the response to antipsychotic drugs might be deficient or insufficient with a low response rate of 30-50%, alongside adverse events in some of the patients (Haddad and Correll, 2018). The response of the organism to the drug used in the treatment of a disease varies between individuals, and genetic factors are determined to be the primary causes underlying the etiology (Lally and MacCabe, 2015). Most of the enzymes metabolizing drugs and xenobiotics have polymorphic gene regions resulting in different levels of enzyme activity between individuals (Guengerich and Cheng, 2011).

CYP2D6 enzyme is the most studied drug-metabolizing enzyme, which is a member of the cytochrome P450 (CYP450) monooxygenase enzyme system, composed of enzymes and generally acts as terminal oxidase in the electron transport chain. The CYP450 family is an enzyme group in the biotransformation process of the drugs. One of the enzymes in this family is the CYP2D6 enzyme group and consists of over 100 different isoenzymes with different affinity to the similar doses of different substrates mainly opiates, neuroleptics, antidepressants, and β-blockers (Ingelman-Sundberg, 2004). The CYP2D6 *3 allele produces an inactive enzyme due to the 2549 A deletion in exon 5 and results in the loss of enzyme function. On the other hand, the CYP2D6 *4 allele produces an inactive enzyme that results from the

1846 G>A substitution in the exon 4 of the gene (Mauri et al., 2014). Risperidone (RSP) and Olanzapine (OLZ) are widely used antipsychotic drugs; the former has potent antagonistic properties for the dopamine D2 and serotonin 5-HT2 receptors, whereas the latter shows antagonist activity for D2/5-HT2, histamine H1 and muscarinic M1 receptors (Qi, Yin, Zhang and Wang, 2020). Sertraline (SRT) is a selective serotonin reuptake inhibitor (SSRI) used in the treatment of mild to moderate depressive symptoms (Santarsieri and Schwartz, 2015).

Antipsychotic and antidepressant drugs show their therapeutic efficiency within a narrow window. Two non-functioning CYP2D6 alleles result in the increased plasma concentration of these drugs contributing to an increased risk of adverse drug reactions and intoxication. Thus, the patient-based genotyping of certain drug-metabolizing enzymes is of concern in order to provide a safe drug dose particularly for the individuals with genetic variations negatively affecting the activity of these enzymes (Lesche, Mostafa, Everall, Pantelis and Bousman, 2020).

The aim of this study is to investigate the pharmacogenetic variations in terms of gene copy numbers, CYP2D6 *3, and *4 single nucleotide polymorphisms (SNPs) among psychiatric patients under treatment with RSP, OLZ and SRT. It was also performed a quantitative study on the levels of these drugs and their metabolites in the urine and blood samples of these individuals.

Materials and Methods

The study included 77 hospitalized and outpatient individuals with an ICD-10 based diagnosis of schizophrenia spectrum disorder or depression, who are drug-naïve in terms of antipsychotics and SSRIs. Blood samples were obtained from 77 patients who were using the drugs containing OLZ, RSP, SRT for the quantitative analysis of the drugs and their metabolites. Simultaneous urine samples were obtained from 39 of 77 individuals in the patient group. Thirty-eight healthy individuals who were not diagnosed with any kind of psychiatric condition and did not use any medication served as the control group. All participants were of Caucasian origin. The clinical and demographic data for the patients and the control group were given in Table 1. All participants provided informed consent and studies were approved by the ethics committee of Istanbul University Cerrahpaşa Medical Faculty (2009/19174).

Three different experimental procedures were applied in the study. First, we performed a melting curve analysis by Real-Time Polymerase Chain Reaction (RT-PCR) to determine the SNPs of CYP2D6 for *3 and *4 alleles after DNA isolation with patient and control blood; and second, expression studies by RT-PCR to determine the CYP2D6 gene copy number. Thirdly, the active substance and/or metabolite concentrations in the blood and urine of patients using the drugs of interest were performed using a Liquid Chromatography-Tandem Mass Spectrometry (LC-MS/MS) based approach.

Table 1. Demographic data of the study group and control subjects

	Patient group (n = 77)	Control group (n = 38)
Gender (Female/Male)	32/45	22/16
Mean age (Min-Max)	37.6 (14-73)	32.7 (20-59)
Alcohol use	11 (14.5%)	N/A
Smoking	37 (48.7%)	N/A
Substance abuse	4 (5.3%)	N/A

Genetic Studies

Genomic DNA was extracted according to the manufacturer's instructions from whole blood samples by the High Pure PCR Template Preparation Kit (Roche, Germany). The isolated genomic DNA samples were stored at 4 °C until further processing.

Genotyping of CYP2D6 *3 (rs35742686, 2549delA) and CYP2D6 *4 (rs3892097, 1846G > A) variants was performed on Roche Light Cycler 480 Real-Time PCR platform (Roche Diagnostics GmbH, Mannheim, Germany). The real-time PCR reactions were carried out in the final volume of 20 μL consisted of 2 μL of Tag Man Genotyping Master Mix (Roche Molecular Systems, Inc.), 4 μL of mixed each forward, reverse, and variant-specific probes (Lightmix), 7.4 μL of nuclease-free water, and 1.6 μL of $MgCl_2$. Thermocycling conditions were as follows: 95 °C for 10 min, followed by 40 cycles of 95 °C for 5 s, 62 °C for 10 s, and 72 °C for 15 s. Positive and negative controls were included in each run.

Required DNA purification was obtained using High Pure PCR Product Purification Kit and single SNP genotyping was performed by using LightCycler FastStart DNA Master HybProbe and LightMix® assay probes (Roche, Germany).

Gene expression study was performed with the probes and primer sequences designed for two regions of the CYP2D6 gene (Intron 6 and Exon 9) and Albumin gene (Intron 12) as an internal reference gene using the LightCycler® TaqMan Master Kit. For the determination of gene expression, the DNA isolates were brought to room temperature. The total volume of the mixture was determined according to the number of samples to be analyzed. The prepared mixture was transferred to 20 μL of LightCycler® capillary tubes on a pre-cooled capillary adapter. In each study, negative control without DNA sample was analyzed for contamination control simultaneously with the samples. The resulting assay results were recorded as Cp (threshold cycle) value, and calculated via albumin as the reference gene. Among the Cp results of the study group, the sample with the lowest albumin expression was selected as "calibrator."

Chromatographic Studies

Blood samples were collected after eight weeks of medication use into Na2-EDTA containing blood collection tubes in the morning hours, 12 h after the bedtime dose, and immediately before the morning dose. Urine samples were collected into NaF2 (5 mg/mL) added sterile plastic collection cups after the blood withdrawal on the same day. Plasma and urine samples were stored at -80 °C until the day of analysis.

Plasma concentrations of OLZ, RSP, SRT, and Paliperidon (PLP) as the major metabolite of RSP were measured by an LC-MS/MS method (Zivak Tandem Gold, Zivac Technologies, FL, USA). The methods were validated for the concentration range 1-50 ng/mL for OLZ, 0.5-100 ng/mL for RSP and PLP, and 5-250 ng/mL for SRT for the plasma samples, whereas linearity was confirmed between 0.5-250 ng/mL for OLZ, RSP, and PLP, and 1-250 ng/mL for SRT for the urine samples. The data on the precision, accuracy, limit of detection (LOD), limit of quantitation (LOQ), and recovery analyses were shown in Table 2.

Compounds were separated using a linear gradient on an analytical reverse phase C18 column (Phenomenex, Luna 3 μ, C18 (2), 100 Å, 150 x 2.00 mm). Mobile phase A was 5 mM acetic acid (pH = 4.5), and mobile phase B consisted of chromatographic purity methanol. The gradient ratio of the mobile phase A was 8%, whereas 92% for the mobile phase B during the 13-min period of the analysis. The flow rate was 0.23 mL/min, and the oven was set at 50 °C.

Table 2. Analytical performance parameters of the LC-MS-MS method for both plasma and urine

		SRT	OLZ	RSP	PLP
Plasma	Calibration ranges (ng/mL)	5-250	1-50	0.5-100	0.5-100
	LOD (ng/mL)	3.59	0.27	0.006	0.019
	LOQ (ng/mL)	11.85	0.89	0.018	0.063
	Recovery % (RSD) (n=11)				
	0.5 ng/mL	*	*	102.5 (7.95)	114.1 (9.01)
	1 ng/mL	*	82.1 (10.19)	*	*
	5 ng/mL	85.7 (7.31)	92.3 (5.79)	*	*
	25 ng/mL	85.4 (9.28)	107.9 (3.22)	104.8 (2.59)	103.0 (3.21)
	100 ng/mL	96.6 (4.24)	*	105.5 (1.46)	100.7 (4.17)
	Between-day Precision (CV%) (n = 3)				
	10 ng/mL	13.94	6.96	7.91	8.83
	25 ng/mL	*	6.07	*	*
	100 ng/mL	4.94	*	1.57	2.18
	Within-day Precision (CV%) (n = 3)				
	10 ng/mL	13.49	2.82	6.58	7.62
	25 ng/mL	*	3.22	*	*
	100 ng/mL	4.24	*	1.47	4.17
	Accuracy (Bias%) (n = 6)				
	10 ng/mL	4.21	9.62	10.71	2.75
	100 ng/mL	3.38	7.99*	5.51	0.78
Urine	Calibration ranges (ng/mL)	1.0-250	0.5-250	0.5-250	0.5-250
	LOD (ng/mL)	3.54	0.06	0.006	0.012
	LOQ (ng/mL)	11.67	0.20	0.020	0.039
	Recovery % (RSD) (n = 5)				
	0.5 ng/mL	*	*	86.6 (12.97)	89.5 (10.81)
	1 ng/mL	*	103.1 (12.00)	*	*
	5 ng/mL	109.6 (6.17)	89.2 (12.19)	*	*
	25 ng/mL	98.7 (3.53)	95.8 (4.95)	105.0 (3.45)	99.5 (3.65)
	100 ng/mL	102.6 (5.32)	80.4 (3.85)	102.5 (5.28)	84.4 (3.60)
	Between-day Precision (CV%) (n = 3)				
	10 ng/mL	6.64	12.49	6.45	12.85
	100 ng/mL	3.57	1.89	2.46	2.98
	Within-day Precision (CV%) (n = 6)				
	10 ng/mL	3.52	10.15	7.12	11.13
	100 ng/mL	5.32	3.85	5.28	3.6
	Accuracy (Bias%) (n = 6)				
	10 ng/mL	7.63	14.86	4.90	8.98
	100 ng/mL	2.64	4.85	2.54	5.66

- Recovery analysis was not performed at this concentration.
- SRT: sertraline, OLZ: olanzapine, RSP: risperidone, PLP: paliperidone

Quantitative analyses of active substance amounts, blood, and urine samples of patients were performed by using automatic LC-MS/MS software (Varian MS Workstation System Control, v.6.9.1) using the calibration curves for each analyte. Samples were diluted 10-fold and quantified when the obtained results exceeded the upper limit of the calibration range. The final elutes which were obtained by the liquid-liquid extraction of collected urine and blood samples were quantified.

500 µL of plasma and 1 mL urine samples after liquid sample preparation at pH = 9.4-10 were mixed with 500 µL eluted with 500 µL including 25 ng/mL of the aqueous internal standard solution (Reboxetine), respectively. Ethyl acetate:n-heptane (2:1) (v/v) mix was used as extraction reagents.

Statistical Analysis

The Hardy-Weinberg equilibrium analysis was performed to compare the observed and expected allele and genotype frequencies of *CYPD6 *3 and *4* by using the chi-square ($\chi 2$) test. The Kolmogorov-Smirnov test was used to test the normal distribution of the data on gene copy numbers. Non-parametric tests were applied to the data when the results showed a skewed pattern. The difference between the patient and the control groups in terms of gene copy numbers were evaluated by the Mann-Whitney U test.

The active drug concentration per dose was compared with the number of CYP2D6 gene copies and CYP2D6 *3 and *4 genotypes. The correlation between these variables was evaluated with Spearman's correlation test.

A *p*-value below 0.05 was considered statistically significant for all statistical calculations. All statistical analyses were performed using Statistical Package for Social Sciences (SPSS) software (version 17, Chicago, USA).

Results

The allele and genotype frequencies of CYP2D6 *3 and *4 alleles and expression profiles of the patient and control group are shown in Table 3. CYP2D6 *3 allele frequencies were equal to the patient and control groups (0.01; $p = 0.609$), whereas the frequency of CYP2D6 *4 is 0.15 in the patient group and 0.04 in the control group (*p < 0.05*).

Twenty-one out of 77 patients (27.2%) in the study group had at least one mutant allele for CYP2D6 *4. Of these, only two patients were homozygous mutants (*4/*4), while the remaining 19 patients were heterozygous (wt/*4). In the control group, three individuals were heterozygous mutant allele carriers for CYP2D6 *4. No homozygosity was observed for CYP2D6 *3 in the patient and the control group. Chi-Square test revealed a significant difference between the patients and the control group in the 90% confidence interval in genotype frequencies of allele *4; ($p<0.1$) while there was no significant difference in genotype frequencies of allele *3 ($p = 0.873$).

Table 3. Genotype and expression pattern of the study group and control samples

Allele	Allele frequency	
	Total number of alleles	
	Patient group (n = 154) (77 x 2)	Control group (n = 76) (38 x 2)
CYP2D6*3	0.01	0.01
CYP2D6*4	0.15	0.04
	Genotype frequency	
	Patient group (n = 77)	Control group (n = 38)
	CYP2D6*3	
*3/*3	0.0 (0/77)	0.0 (0/38)
*3/wt	0.013 (1/77)	0.026 (1/38)
wt/wt	0.987 (76/77)	0.974 (37/38)
	CYP2D6*4	
*4/*4	0.026 (2/77)	0.0 (0/38)
*4/wt	0.247 (19/77)	0.079 (3/38)
wt/wt	0.727 (56/77)	0.921 (35/38)
	Expression analysis*	
	CYP2D6 Intron 6	
$R = 0.5$	18	-
$R = 1.0$	38	23
$R = 1.5$	10	-
$R \geq 2.0$	11	4
	CYP2D6 Exon 9	
$R = 0.5$	36	4
$R = 1.0$	25	16
$R = 1.5$	8	2
$R \geq 2.0$	8	5

* The number of subjects in the control group for expression analysis is 27.
$R=0.5$ (Gene number is 1, or gene activity is low).
$R=1$ (Gene number is 2).
$R= 1.5$ (Gene number is 3).
$R \geq 2.0$ (Gene number is ≥ 4).

The number of gene copies for exon 9 in the patient group was significantly lower than the 95% confidence interval when compared to the control group ($p < 0.05$). The difference between gene copy numbers for intron 6 was not significant ($p = 0.376$) (df = 102). The correlation between gene copy numbers obtained from intron 6 and exon 9 regions was analyzed by nonparametric Spearman's correlation test and a significant correlation was found at a 95% confidence interval ($p < 0.05$).

Table 4. Analyte concentrations and analyte/dose ratios in the plasma and urine samples of the patient group

Sample type	Analyte	Mean ± SD	Min	Max	Median
Plasma (ng/mL)	SRT (n = 2)	11.9 ± 0.07	11.9	12.0	11.95
	OLZ (n = 21)	41.0 ± 36.8	LOQ	147.3	31.5
	RSP (n = 17)	5.34 ± 3.7	LOQ	110	4.0
	PLP (n = 17)	17.9 ± 10.7	LOQ	37.4	14.6
Urine (ng/mL)	SRT (n = 2)	57.3±14.1	47.3	67.3	57.3
	OLZ (n = 19)	294.2 ± 264.0	LOQ	976.9	320.0
	RSP (n = 16)	92.1 ± 104.4	LOQ	297.5	55.6
	PLP (n = 16)	585.7 ± 687.8	LOQ	2084.0	308.0
Plasma (ng/mL)	OLZ/D	3.26 ± 2.42	0.1	9.4	3.15
	PLP/RSP	4.64 ± 2.68	0.4	8.4	5.15
	(PLP/RSP)/D	1.05 ± 0.96	0.1	2.8	0.55
	SRT/D	0.1 ± 0	0.1	0.1	0.1
Urine (ng/mL)	OLZ/D	22.62 ± 22.06	1.1	70.0	16.0
	PLP/RSP	19.28 ± 23.42	0.2	86.2	11.1
	(PLP/RSP)/D	8.57 ± 23.39	0.1	86.2	1.7
	SRT/D	0.6 ± 0.14	0.5	0.7	0.6

Abbreviations: OLZ/D: Olanzapine concentration/Dose; PLP/RSP: Paliperidone/Risperidone concentration; (PLP/RSP)/D: (Paliperidone/Risperidone concentration)/Dose; SRT/D: Sertraline concentration/Dose; SD: Standard deviation.

Table 5. Statistical analysis of the drug concentration/dose ratio of the patients according to presence of the CYP2D6*4 allele

C/D (ng/mL)	Mean (Non-CYP2D6*4 carriers)	Mean (CYP2D6*4 carriers)	P value	SD
OLZ/D (Urine)	19.77	25.52	0.635	16
OLZ/D (Plasma)	3.02	3.98	0.458	16
(PLP/RSP)/D (Urine)	9.01	0.825	0.522	14
(PLP/RSP)/D (Plasma)	0.769	0.125	0.291	15

Abbreviations: OLZ/D: Olanzapine concentration/Dose; PLP/RSP: Paliperidone/Risperidone concentration; (PLP/RSP)/D: (Paliperidone/Risperidone concentration)/Dose; SRT/D: Sertraline concentration/Dose; SD: Standard deviation.

LC-MS/MS analysis on the amounts of active substances in 39 patients and drug concentrations (C/D) per dose were shown in Table 4. There was no significant difference in substance concentration between the groups carrying the mutant or wildtype CYP2D6 *4 alleles ($p > 0.05$) (Table 5).

Conclusion

The CYP2D6 gene copy number allows accurate estimation of the CYP2D6 phenotype when used in combination with SNP genotyping (Fang et al., 2014). Individuals with low enzyme activities may experience serious adverse drug reactions and may experience insufficient therapeutic efficacy (Alomar, 2014). In addition to CYP2D6 genotyping, gene copy number determination is essential to determine the correct phenotype (Wigmore et al., 2020). Since psychiatric drugs are the most common drugs in intoxication cases, the polymorphisms of CYP2D6, which is the major enzyme that metabolizes these drugs, are of great importance in clinical and forensic sciences while evaluating adverse effects in patients treated with these agents.

In our study, we evaluated the gene expression level in the exon 9 and intron 6 gene regions by using the TaqMan RT-PCR method and calculated the number of gene copies. We found a significant difference between the patients and the control group in the number of exon 9 gene copies. We also found a significant difference between the patient and control groups for the *4 allele by melting curve analysis. The fact that the frequency of the patient group *4 was significantly higher than that of the control group indicated that the incidence of poor metabolizers was higher between psychiatric patients and that the risk of adverse drug reactions might be higher when one or more active drug agents were used in the treatment.

In their study with 110 volunteers, Chiurillo et al., found the total frequency of CYP2D6 enzyme metabolizing alleles as 19.5% in a Venezuelan population (Chiurillo, Grimán, Morán, Camargo and Ramírez, 2009). Andreassen et al., reported that 18% of the patients with schizophrenia carry *4 alleles, whereas the frequency of the *3 allele was 0.5% in this group. They further stated that 5 out of 100 patients had CYP2D6 *4/*4 phenotype, suggesting that these patients experienced a higher frequency of side effects than others, and these side effects showed a permanent state with the intake of antipsychotic drugs (Andreassen, MacEwan, Gulbrandsen, McCreadie and Steen, 1997). In our study, we found that 15% of our study group had CYP2D6

*4, 1% had CYP2D6 *3 alleles, and the number of CYP2D6 *4/*4 among 77 patients was 2 (2.6%).

Kawanishi et al., found that 81 out of 108 patients with a mood disorder and resistant to antidepressant treatment, and 10% of them had gene duplication (Kawanishi, Lundgren, Agren and Bertilsson, 2004). The frequency in their study group was significantly different from the prevalence of 0.8-1.0% in the normal population, suggesting that gene duplication is a possible cause of continuous mood disorder. In our study, we performed a relative calculation of the number of gene copies and found that more than 20% of the patients had ≥2 gene copies. However, a complicated methodological approach including Long-PCR or additional methods to identify the other alleles is required in order to reveal the active genes on these gene duplication sites.

In the analyses of CYP2D6 *3 and *4 genotypes and gene copy numbers by melting curve and gene expression studies, we observed deviations in some of the individuals in the patient group. It should be taken into account that we determined only the polymorphism of *3 and *4 alleles in the context of our study, however, considering that the CYP2D6 gene has more than 100 alleles and two pseudogenes it is possible that the genotype result of each patient does not exactly match the number of gene copies. In addition, the possibility of the presence of a hybrid gene should be considered. On the other hand, factors affecting enzyme induction and inhibition might be other causes of this deviation. In the simultaneous administration of multiple drugs, the concentration of the drugs' active ingredients in the circulation may change as one of the other active ingredients causes enzyme inhibition or induction (Palleria et al., 2013).

In our study, we compared the mean concentrations of OLZ and RSP active substances per dose in the blood and urine of patients with and without the CYP2D6 *4 allele. Although we did not find any statistically significant difference in blood and urine levels for both substances, the difference between them might be remarkable. The OLZ/D (OLZ/dose) values were higher in patients carrying the CYP2D6 *4 alleles, suggesting that the active substance OLZ is metabolized more slowly. In contrast, the metabolite/active substance ratio comparison in blood and urine samples for PLP/RSP suggests that RSP active substance is metabolized more slowly in CYP2D6 *4 allele carriers. However, the findings did not show a statistical significance, possibly due to the limited number of patients.

In a study with 122 children and adolescent subjects, Theisen et al., found plasma OLZ concentration/dose (C/D) ratio in the interval of 0.8-5.5 ng/mL, with a mean value of 2.6 ng/mL (Theisen et al., 2006). In our study group, the C/D interval was between 0.29-9.4 ng/mL for plasma, and 1.07 and 70.0 ng/mL for urine samples, with mean values of 3.25 ng/mL and 19.23 ng/mL, respectively. Differences between two study groups might be a result of genetic mutations or expression rates of the enzymes in the selected patient group; or the level of a psychiatric condition, age, or other concomitant medications. It is reported that C/D ratio is 38% higher in patients treated with other medications alongside OLZ when compared with OLZ monotherapy (Theisen et al., 2006). Herken et al., reported that efficient systemic levels cannot be maintained in approximately 10% of patients, and severe side effects may be observed in 1-2% due to toxic levels of active ingredients when an antipsychotic or antidepressant drug metabolized by CYP2D6 enzyme is prescribed to Turkish patients (Herken, Aynacıoğlu, Esgi and Vırıt, 2001). According to the results of our study, since 15% of psychiatric patients using antipsychotic and antidepressant drugs metabolized by CYP2D6 carry at least one poor metabolizing allele, and these patients are more likely to have adverse effects, the determination of CYP2D6 enzyme activity of an individual before the use of antipsychotics and antidepressant drugs might be beneficial in predicting the efficiency and possible adverse effects (Arranz et al., 2019).

The number of patients using sertraline was limited to two in our study group. We found that both patients treated with a daily dose of 100 mg, and had a mutation for the CYP2D6 *4 allele being intermediate metabolizers. When we analyzed the gene expression patterns, the gene expression level in exon 9 was lower in the patient with a higher urine SRT level. Since both patients were male and, with a similar age of 26 and 28 years, excluding age and gender-related factors, we suggest that the difference in urine-sertraline levels between these two patients might be due to the slower enzyme rate of the enzyme, the amount of substance excreted without metabolization is higher in the patient with lower expression level. Thus, the similar plasma SRT levels in two patients might be explained as a drug concentration in the steady-state, depending on the regular intake of SRT containing medication.

According to a study conducted in Australia between the years 2002 and 2008, 381 out of 1123 deaths between these years were drug-related; whereas 28 were directly related to serotonin toxicity, raising the question of whether these cases are poor metabolizers for these drugs (Pilgrim, Gerostamoulos and Drummer, 2010).

Psychiatric patients a special group, and may be under the treatment with agents for long years, they are at risk for adverse effects caused by these drugs in the short or long term, and the risk might increase while other drug active substances are added in the therapy. The findings of our study also reveal that at least 20% of the patients have high expression of the CYP2D6 gene, and they will be exposed to the side effects of active metabolite in case of prolonged treatment periods. Furthermore, the effective dose cannot be provided in these patients in case of a pro-drug containing treatment (Bousman and Hopwood, 2016).

Our study undertook an LC-MS/MS system-based approach with the development of an analytical method with high accuracy and low measurement limits. To our knowledge, this is the first study evaluating the CYP2D6 gene copy numbers, CYP2D6 *3, and *4 allele expressions and the concentrations of drugs and metabolites metabolized by this enzyme in biological samples, simultaneously.

We observed that the previously described 5% of CYP2D6 *4 allele frequency was 15% in psychiatric patients, emphasizing the importance of drug-metabolizing enzyme polymorphisms in special populations in order to acquire an efficient treatment. Detecting the polymorphism ratio of the CYP2D6 enzyme in the specific populations and reviewing the treatment doses would contribute to more effective and cost-effective management of the diseases, and the adverse effects caused by interpersonal differences that may lead to death would be overcome.

Conflict of Interest

The authors declare no conflict of interest.

Acknowledgments

Authors would like to thank to Scientific Research Fund of Istanbul University-Cerrahpasa for support of this study with the project number 4764. Authors also grateful to the staff of the psychiatry clinic in Istanbul University-Cerrahpaşa, Medical Faculty, Department of Psychiatry and Department of Microbiology for their cooperation.

References

Alomar, M. J. Factors affecting the development of adverse drug reactions (rReview article). *Saudi Pharm J.* 2014, 22(2), 83-94. doi: 10.1016/j.jsps.2013.02.003.

Andreassen, O. A, MacEwan, T., Gulbrandsen, A. K., McCreadie, R. G., Steen, V. M. Non-functional CYP2D6 alleles and risk for neuroleptic-induced movement disorders in schizophrenic patients. *Psychopharmacology* 1997, 131 (2), 174-9. DOI: 10.1007/s002130050281

Arranz, M. J., Gonzalez-Rodriguez, A., Perez-Blanco, J., Penadés, R., Gutierrez, B., Ibañez, L., Arias, B., Brunet, M., Cervilla, J., Salazar, J., and Catalan, R., A pharmacogenetic intervention for the improvement of the safety profile of antipsychotic treatments. *Transl Psychiatry.* 2019, 9(1), 177. doi: 10.1038/s41398-019-0511-9.

Bousman, C. A., Hopwood, M. Commercial pharmacogenetic-based decision-support tools in psychiatry. *Lancet Psychiatry* 2016, 3, 585–590. DOI: 10.1016/S2215-0366(16)00017-1.

Butler, M. G. Pharmacogenetics and Psychiatric Care: A Review and Commentary. *J Ment Health Clin. Psychol.* 2018, 2(2), 17-24.

Chiurillo, M. A., Grimán, P., Morán, Y., Camargo, M. E., Ramírez, J. L. Analysis of CYP2D6 gene variation in Venezuelan population: Implications for forensic toxicology. *Forensic Science International: Genetics Supplement Series* 2009, 2, 483-484. https://doi.org/ 10.1016/j.fsigss.2009.08.044.

Fang, H., Liu, X., Ramírez, J., Choudhury, N., Kubo, M., Im, H. K., Konkashbaev, A., Cox, N. J., Ratain, M. J., Nakamura, Y., O'Donnell, P. H. Establishment of CYP2D6 reference samples by multiple validated genotyping platforms. *Pharmacogenomics J.* 2014, 14(6), 564-72. doi: 10.1038/tpj.2014.27.

Guengerich, F. P., Cheng, Q. Orphans in the human cytochrome P450 superfamily: approaches to discovering functions and relevance in pharmacology. *Pharmacol. Rev.* 2011, 63(3), 684-99. doi: 10.1124/pr.110.003525.

Haddad, P. M., Correll, C. U. The acute efficacy of antipsychotics in schizophrenia: a review of recent meta-analyses. *Ther Adv. Psychopharmacol.* 2018, 8(11), 303-318. doi: 10.1177/2045125318781475.

Herken, H., Aynacıoğlu, Ş., Esgi, K., Vırıt, O. Psikiyatri Hastalarında Sitokrom P450 2D6 Yavaş ve Ultra Hızlı Metabolizör Sıklıkları [Slow and Ultra Fast Metabolizer Frequencies]. *Türk Psikiyatri. Dergisi.* 2001, 12(2), 83-88.

Ingelman-Sundberg, M. Pharmacogenetics of cytochrome P450 and its applications in drug therapy: the past, present and future. *Trends Pharm. Sci.* 2004, 25, 193–200. DOI: 10.1016/j.tips.2004.02.007

Kawanishi, C., Lundgren, S., Agren, H., Bertilsson, L. Increased incidence of CYP2D6 gene duplication in patients with persistent mood disorders: ultrarapid metabolism of antidepressants as a cause of nonresponse. A pilot study. *Eur. J. Clin. Pharmacol.* 2004, 59, 803-807. DOI: 10.1007/s00228-003-0701-4

Lally, J., MacCabe, J. H. Antipsychotic medication in schizophrenia: a review. *Br. Med. Bull.* 2015, 114(1), 169-79. doi: 10.1093/bmb/ldv017.

Lesche, D., Mostafa, S., Everall, I., Pantelis, C., Bousman, C. A. Impact of CYP1A2, CYP2C19, and CYP2D6 genotype- and phenoconversion-predicted enzyme activity on clozapine exposure and symptom severity. *Pharmacogenomics J.* 2020, 20(2), 192-201 doi: 10.1038/s41397-019-0108-y.

Lin, J. H. Pharmacokinetic and Pharmacodynamic Variability: A Daunting Challenge in Drug Therapy. *Current Drug Metabolism* 2007, 8, 109. https://doi.org/10.2174/138920007779816002

Mauri, M. C., Paletta, S., Maffini, M., Colasanti, A., Dragogna, F., Di Pace, C., Altamura, A. C. Clinical pharmacology of atypical antipsychotics: an update. *EXCLI J.* 2014, 13, 1163-91.

Palleria, C., Di Paolo, A., Giofrè, C., Caglioti, C., Leuzzi, G., Siniscalchi, A., De Sarro, G., Gallelli, L. Pharmacokinetic drug-drug interaction and their implication in clinical management. *J. Res. Med. Sci.* 2013, 18(7), 601-10. PMID: 24516494; PMCID: PMC 3897029.

Pilgrim, J. L., Gerostamoulos D, Drummer OH. Deaths involving serotonergic drugs, *Forensic Science International* 2010, 198, 110-117. DOI: 10.1016/j.forsciint.2010.01.014

Qi, G., Yin, S., Zhang, G., Wang X. Genetic and epigenetic polymorphisms of eNOS and CYP2D6 in mainland Chinese Tibetan, Mongolian, Uygur, and Han populations. *Pharmacogenomics J.* 2020, 20, 114–125.

Santarsieri, D., Schwartz, T. L. Antidepressant efficacy and side-effect burden: a quick guide for clinicians. *Drugs Context.* 2015, 4, 212290. doi: 10.7573/dic.212290.

Theisen, F. M., Haberhausen, M., Schulz, E., Fleischhaker, C., Clement, H. W., Heinzel-Gutenbrunner, M., et al., Serum levels of olanzapine and its N-desmethyl and 2-hydroxymethyl metabolites in child and adolescent psychiatric disorders: effects of dose, diagnosis, age, sex, smoking, and comedication. *Ther. Drug Monit.* 2006, 28, 750-759. DOI: 10.1097/01.ftd.0000249950.75462.7f

Wigmore, E. M., Hafferty, J. D., Hall, L. S., Howard, D. M., Clarke, T. K., Fabbri, C., et al., Genome-wide association study of antidepressant treatment resistance in a population-based cohort using health service prescription data and meta-analysis with GENDEP. *Pharmacogenomics J.* 2020, 20(2), 329-341. doi: 10.1038/s41397-019-0067-3.

Chapter 4

Old Benzodiazepine, New NPS−Phenazepam: A Method Development Study

Merve Kuloglu Genc[1,*], MSc
and James Barker[2], PhD

[1] Presently at Institute of Forensic Sciences and Legal Medicine,
Istanbul University- Cerrahpaşa, Istanbul, Turkey
[2] School of Life Sciences, Pharmacy and Chemistry, Kingston University,
Kingston-Upon-Thames, London, UK

Abstract

Designer benzodiazepines are a novel type of new psychoactive substance (NPS), often known as NPS-benzodiazepines. They are especially harmful, owing to inadequate toxicity information and a tendency to consider them as therapeutic drugs, which may result in misdiagnosis, treatment with consequent severe adverse effects and occasionally death. Phenazepam is a frequently abused, long-acting benzodiazepine, which has recently been categorized as a NPS-benzodiazepine. Phenazepam has been released into the recreational drug market from time to time for many years, but its reappearance as a NPS-benzodiazepine has demanded a cost-effective, easy and reliable analytical method for accurate identification and quantification of this substance for forensic and clinical purposes. This paper presents, a validated method specific to phenazepam using reverse-phase-high-performance-liquid chromatography coupled to ultraviolet - visible spectrophotometric detection. The proposed method analysed phenazepam within 2 minutes, accomplishing an overall 102.63 ± 0.06% accuracy, 0.220% intraday and 0.008% inter-day precision. The limit of

---

[*] Corresponding Author's Email: merve.kuloglu@iuc.edu.tr.

In: The Dangers of Psychoactive Substances
Editor: Denise J. Burton
ISBN: 979-8-88697-705-9
© 2023 Nova Science Publishers, Inc.

detection and limit of quantitation values were determined as 0.158 and 0.526 µg/mL, respectively. The validated method was also successfully applied to a spiked hair sample. The validation performance of the developed method was satisfactory considering international council on harmonisation guidelines.

Keywords: Phenazepam, Benzodiazepine, NPS, NPS-benzodiazepine, HPLC

Introduction

Benzodiazepines (BZD) are commonly used psychotherapeutic drugs that have a significant number of group members, which are typically prescribed for the treatments of anxiety, epilepsy, insomnia, alcohol withdrawal and post-traumatic stress disorders due to their sedative and hypnotic effects. Their easy accessibility and high demand in the pharmaceutical industry make BZD convenient target for illegal drug producers (EMCDDA, 2021).

Phenazepam [7-bromo-5-(2-chlorophenyl)-1,3-dihydro-2H-1,4-benzo-diazepin-2-one] is a 1,4-benzodiazepine group member (Figure 1) with common street names bonsai, fenaz and Soviet benzo. It possesses similar effects with the rest of the BZD family by creating central nervous system (CNS) depression, so its most usual treatment areas are muscle relaxing, anxiety, insomnia, alcohol withdrawal, epilepsy, and panic attacks. The substance has a relatively long half-life, up to 60 hours, making phenazepam a long-acting drug. Loss in balance, impaired vision, slurred speech, amnesia, and CNS depression are all common side effects (EMCDDA 2021; UN CND 2016; WHO 2015). However, what makes phenazepam dangerous is its long-lasting effects, which causes users to believe the dosage that they had was insufficient, leading to overdose and in some cases, death. Additionally, the benzodiazepine family is known for its use with other substances to heighten and prolong the high or to ease the withdrawal effects of the other drugs (Vogel et al., 2013). Similar to other BZD, when phenazepam is used in combination with substances acting on the CNS such as alcohol, opioids or synthetic cannabinoids, the situation becomes life threatening (Shearer et al., 2015).

From the early 2000s, a new group of psychoactive substance, called new psychoactive substances (NPS) has emerged on the drug market and they were promoted as "legal highs" to increase their demand. In addition to newly manufactured drugs in this group, previously produced substances that have not been seen on the market for some time are reintroduced in the same form or with minor chemical modifications in order to circumvent the law EMCDDA 2021; Moosmann and Auwärter 2018). The most dangerous aspects of these substances are that they contain a large number of psychoactive substances and by-products in their content. Many of these NPS-benzodiazepines have never been subjected to the clinical testing that licensed drugs must undergo. As a result, the rising availability of these NPS-benzodiazepines creates major health threats to poly-drug users, misusers and benzodiazepine-dependent individuals who are unable to receive their prescription and must seek benzodiazepines from other sources (Manchester et al., 2018). This situation leads to the inability to predict short and long-term clinical damages and becomes challenging for emergency physicians and forensic toxicologists, especially, when substances that do not have much toxicological information even on their own, are released in mixtures (Gerostamoulos et al., 2016).

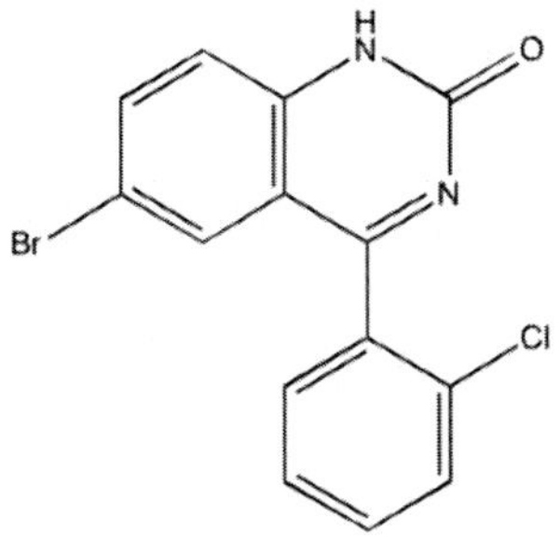

Figure 1. The chemical structure of phenazepam.

In 2007, the European monitoring centre for drugs and drug addiction (EMCDDA) reported the first illicit benzodiazepines discovered in Europe as phenazepam (fenazepam) and nimetazepam (EMCDDA-Europol 2007). After numerous "driving under the influence of drugs" (DUID) cases and post mortem findings containing phenazepam, between 2008-2012, many Scandinavian countries (Norway, Sweden and Finland) and United Kingdom (UK) designated phenazepam as a controlled drug (UK scheduled as a Class C drug under the Misuse of Drugs Act 1971) (WHO 2015). However, before being criminalized, it was offered as a "legal high" and was available over the Internet and in "head shops" (Shearer et al., 2015). According to Scottish national drug related death database, phenazepam was the most prevalent BZD involved in NPS-related deaths (23 out of 24 cases) in 2012 (McAuley et al., 2015). Moreover, against all legal efforts, it has been identified in considerable amounts in seized NPS and/or post-mortem results in past years (Shearer et al., 2015; McAuley et al., 2015; Bailey et al., 2010). Recently, phenazepam has also been encountered as a by-product (amongst others) in fake diazepam tablets in Europe and in Erimin-5 tablets (used instead of nimetazepam) in Malaysia and Singapore (Lim et al., 2017).

Phenazepam is released into the illicit drug market for many years, now it's appearance as NPS-benzodiazepines has now demanded easy, rapid and reliable analytical methods for accurate identification and quantification in forensic and clinical settings. Various instruments have been used in forensic and pharmaceutical analysis e.g., liquid chromatography-tandem mass spectroscopy (LC-MS/MS) (Shearer et al., 2015; Crichton et al., 2015; Madry, Kraemer, and Baumgartner 2020; Pettersson, Helander, and Beck 2016; Stephenson, Golz and Brasher 2013), high performance liquid chromatography (HPLC) (Lim et al., 2017; Park et al., 2013) (coupled to ultraviolet-visible spectrophotometry (UV-Vis), gas chromatography-mass spectroscopy (GC-MS) (Bailey et al., 2010; Dargan et al., 2013; Kriikku et al., 2012), thin-layer chromatography (Belova et al., 2018), immunoassays (Kerrigan, Brady-Mellon, and Hinners 2013; Reschly-Krasowski and Krasowski 2018) for detection, however, one of the most widely available techniques in clinical and forensic laboratory settings is HPLC. Phenazepam analysis can be achieved in various matrices, depending on the need and availability often blood, urine and seized materials are preferred. Although hair samples are not frequently encountered in these analyses, hair samples are proven to be credible witnesses specifically for long-term exposure to drugs in clinical and forensic investigations to understand acute and chronic toxicities.

The presented study focused on developing and validating an analytical method for the rapid, cost-effective, and sensitive analysis of phenazepam using HPLC-UV/Vis and to examine the performance of the method on authentic hair samples.

Method and Experimental

Chemicals and Equipment

The reference standard of phenazepam was purchased from LGC (Teddington, UK). HiPerSolv HPLC-grade (99.9% purity) acetonitrile (ACN) was purchased from VWR Chemicals (Leicestershire, UK). AnalaR NORMAPUR methanol (MeOH) was obtained from VWR Chemicals (Leicestershire, UK). Distilled water was obtained from an Elga Water Purifier Unit with DV25 Dock (15 M Ω, High Wycombe, UK). A syringe filter with 0.45 μm pore size was provided from Merck Millipore (Tullagreen, Carrigtwohill, Ireland). VWR Ultrasonic bath was acquired from VWR Chemicals (Leicestershire, UK). A local hairdresser provided the human hair that was utilised in the procedure's development and validation.

Instrumentation

The analytical method was developed using a Varian ProStar HPLC coupled with Varian ProStar 325 UV/Vis detector. The analyte was separated using a SphereClone™ 5 μm ODS (2) 80 A, 150 x 4.6 mm purchased from Phenomenex (Torrance, CA, USA).

To confirm that hair samples were spiked with phenazepam and did not contain the substance at the beginning, Agilent GC operated with MS detector was used. Hair samples incubated in methanol and spiked hair samples were analysed by GC-MS for identification purposes. The column used was DB-1MS; 30 m x 0.25 mm x 0.25 μm and carrier gas was Helium. The split ratio was 20:1 and injection volume was 1 μL. The inlet temperature was 280 °C with a mass scan range 30-550 amu.

Sample Preparation

A stock solution was prepared at a concentration of 1000 μg/mL in MeOH. The solution was sonicated in an ultrasonic bath for 15 min. Working solutions were prepared by diluting the stock solution with MeOH in the range of 1000, 400, 100, 50, 10, 5 and 1 μg/mL. Finally, working solutions were transferred into vials for further HPLC analysis. All stock and working solutions were stored in refrigerator at –18 °C during the study.

Method Development

To achieve an optimum method for phenazepam, different analytical columns (Waters Spherisorb S5 C8, 4.6 x 150 mm; Phenomenex, SphereClone 5 μm

ODS (2), 150 x 4.6 mm), mobile phase percentages (ACN: Water, 90:10, 80:20, 70:30 v/v), flow rates (0.5, 1 and 2 mL/min) and injection volumes were applied until a good gaussian-shaped peak with reasonable retention time was obtained. The optimized method was achieved by using an isocratic elution method, and the details are shown in the Table 1.

Table 1. Optimized analytical method conditions

Mobile phase	20% Water- 80% ACN
Injection volume	10.0 µL
Flow rate	1.00 mL/min
Column temperature	40.00 °C
Detection wavelength	240 nm
Column type	SphereClone 5µm ODS (2), 150 x 4.6 mm

Sample Preparation for Hair Analysis

Sample preparation was conducted by following the society of hair (SOHT) testing guidelines (Cooper, Kronstrand, and Kintz 2012). Hair samples were washed to remove dust, chemical treatments, and other potential external contaminants. Samples were washed twice with water, acetone, and dichloromethane for 2 minutes and sonicated 5 minutes then air-dried. Dried samples were cut into 1 mm segments. Four sets of 50 mg hair samples were weighed out. Then, all sample sets except blank were spiked at 3 different concentrations 1000 (high), 100 (medium) and 10 µg/mL (low). Then, analytes were extracted by incubating for 3 hours in methanol at 37 °C and centrifugation for 15 minutes at 2.300 rcf. After 1 mL of extraction solvent was removed for evaporation under nitrogen at 35 °C. The extracts were reconstituted in methanol and transferred into vials for HPLC analysis.

Method Validation

The proposed analytical method was validated according to the international conference on harmonization (ICH) guidelines in terms of sensitivity, linearity, accuracy, precision, the limit of detection and the limit of quantitation (ICH 2019).
  The lack of interference in the same chromatographic window was used to determine the selectivity of the method. Linearity studies were conducted

by analysing standard solutions in the range of 1-100 μg/mL in triplicates. A five-point calibration curve plotted as concentration against mean peak area was generated using linear regression analysis. The correlation coefficient, slope, and intercept of the calibration curve were calculated. The accuracy and precision studies were evaluated by calculating the recovery, standard deviation (SD) and relative standard deviation (RSD%) values at three concentrations levels 10, 50 and 100 μg/mL (low, medium, high) and three replicates of each concentration. For repeatability (intraday precision), the method was assessed in a short period of time by repeating the experiments three times at 10, 50 and 100 μg/mL (low, medium, high) concentrations. For intermediate precision (inter-day precision), analyses were performed under the same conditions through two consecutive days and three consecutive runs on each day and the results were compared. LOD was determined according to signal to noise ratio as 3:1, representing the lowest quantity of analyte that can be detected with the optimized method. As for LOQ, the signal to noise ratio should be 10:1 for an analyte to be quantitated.

Results and Discussion

Method Development for HPLC

The influence of particular parameters such as peak symmetry and reasonable length of run, was evaluated to obtain better resolution. For this research, a gradient mode was not chosen because it is generally used for separation of complex compounds, which is not the case in this study. Also, due to its drawback of demanding column equilibration prior to each analysis, the isocratic mode was chosen. Two different analytical columns were assessed. Initially, the Waters Spherisorb S5 C8, 4.6 x 150 mm column, which is a reversed phase column, was used. However, due to high pressure problems, tailing and long elution time, the column was changed to a SphereClone 5 μm ODS (2), 150 x 4.6 mm, which is a highly non-polar (hydrophobic) reversed-phase column with 18 carbon chain. This column change reduced the retention time, generated useful pressure values, and helped to obtain better-shaped peaks. Reduced elution time can be chemically explained by making the stationary phase more non-polar, interaction between polar compound (phenazepam) and stationary phase reduces, so that elution will be much faster. Finally, mobile phase composition was changed to obtain sharper peaks for the compound; it was observed that as the ACN composition increased from 40% to 80%, peaks became sharper and clearer, so the retention time became shorter. For this experiment, 80% ACN / 20% water mobile phase composition was found to be the most suitable. Wavelength detection of 240 nm was determined by scanning three concentrations of standard solution (1000, 400, and 100 µg/mL) at 200–400 nm. Figure 2 represents the chromatogram of phenazepam using the optimised HPLC method eluting at 2.17 min.

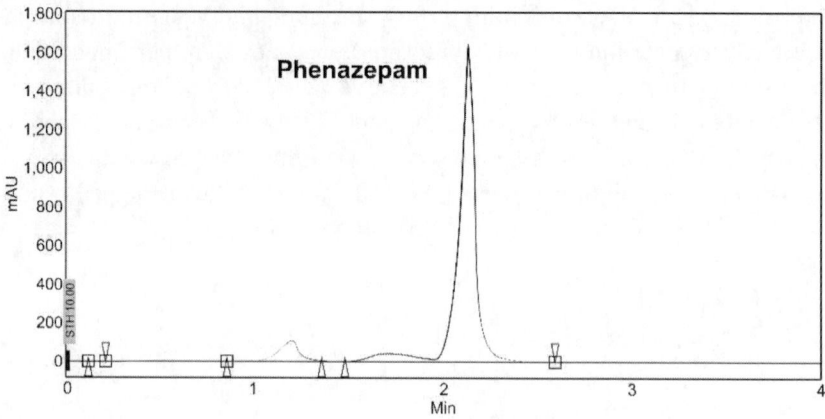

Figure 2. Chromatogram of 100 µg/mL concentrated phenazepam by HPLC using optimized method.

HPLC Method Validation

Linearity

The linearity range was determined as ranging from 1 to 100 µg/mL. All results are shown in Table 2 with their corresponding peak area and SD values.

Peak areas were plotted against phenazepam concentrations to produce a calibration curve. The calibration graph showed that linearity was satisfactory with a 0.9993 (r) correlation coefficient at concentrations ranging from 100 to 1 µg/mL. Based on linear regression calculations, the equation obtained was as follows:

$$y = 555.94 \, x + 2.8989,$$

where the slope is 555.94 and intercept is 2.8989.

Table 2. Measurements of calibration points and their corresponding peak area values

Concentration (µg/mL) (n=3)	Peak area (mAU x min.)	Mean peak area (mAU x min.)	SD
100	58.27 58.30 58.26	58.30	0.02
50	31.12 31.17 30.98	31.10	0.09
10	19.48 19.41 19.36	19.40	0.06
5	6.81 6.87 6.83	6.80	0.03
1	2.27 2.25 2.26	2.30	0.01

SD: Standard Deviation.

Accuracy

Three concentration levels were assessed in terms of recovery involving low (10 µg/mL), medium (50 µg/mL), and high (100 µg/mL), as shown in Table 3. Overall accuracy was measured between 99.65-106.80%, indicating satisfactory results.

Table 3. Accuracy results for optimised HPLC method

Concentration (µg/mL) (n=3)	Peak area (mAU x min.)	Mean peak area (mAU x min.)	Measured concentration (µg/mL)	Recovery %	SD	RSD%
100	58.30 58.26 58.27	58.28	99	99.65	0.021	0.036
50	30.98 31.17 31.12	31.09	51	101.44	0.099	0.318
10	19.48 19.41 19.36	19.42	11	106.80	0.049	0.255
Mean values				102.63	0.056	0.203

RSD: Relative Standard Deviation; SD: Standard Deviation.

Precision

Repeatability (Intra-day precision): The method was evaluated by performing the same analyses three times at three different concentrations in the same day. The results presented in Table 4 were in agreement with the limits established by ICH (ICH 2019).

Table 4. Intra-day precision / repeatability results for optimised HPLC method

Concentration (µg/mL)	Number of analysis	Peak area (mAU x min.)	Mean peak area (mAU x min.)	RSD%
100	1	58.30	58.27	0.036
	2	58.26		
	3	58.27		
50	1	30.98	31.09	0.315
	2	31.17		
	3	31.12		
10	1	19.48	19.43	0.308
	2	19.41		
	3	19.36		
Mean RSD %				0.220

RSD: Relative Standard Deviation.

Intermediate precision (Inter-day precision): Intermediate precision studies carried out in two different days were presented in Table 5. The mean of two inter-day RSD % values was calculated as 0.008%. Due to low RSD % results, it can be said that method successfully satisfied the intermediate precision step.

Limit of Detection (LOD) and Limit of Quantitation (LOQ)

The LOD was found to be 0.158 µg/mL, where LOQ was 0.526 µg/mL. The LOD and LOQ values were found to be appropriate for the clinical and forensic detection of phenazepam from various matrices and seized materials.

Table 5. Inter-day / intermediate precision results for optimised HPLC method

Day	Concentration (µg/mL) (n=3)	Peak area (mAU x min.)	Mean peak area (mAU x min.)	RSD%
1	50	30.74	30.95	0.012
		30.75		
		31.37		
2	50	30.98	31.09	0.003
		31.17		
		31.12		

RSD: Relative Standard Deviation.

Application to Authentic Hair Samples

To prove that hair samples did not contain Phenazepam prior to analysis, firstly, blank hair samples that were extracted with MeOH were analysed by GC-MS. Then, blank and spiked hair samples at three different concentrations, low (10 μg/mL), medium (50 μg/mL), and high (100 μg/mL) were analysed by the validated HPLC method (see Figure 3).

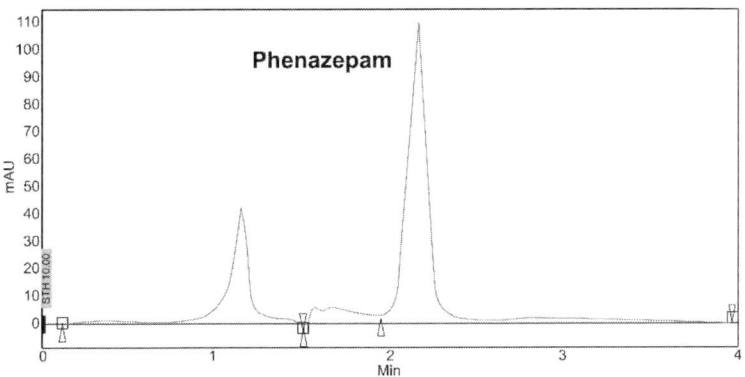

Figure 3. Chromatogram of spiked hair sample at 100 μg/mL.

Phenazepam was quantified and identified with the validated method based upon the retention time in chromatograms. In addition, further confirmation was performed with GC-MS as well and the results obtained shown in Figures 4 and 5. These outcomes suggested the success of the extraction technique used as well as the suitability of the validated method to assess phenazepam in hair samples. The results of the recovery studies based on the extraction of external spiking are presented in the Table 6, demonstrating acceptable outcomes.

It is known that hair samples are reliable witnesses for understanding acute and chronic exposure in clinical and forensic investigations. For this reason, it is important to demonstrate the utility of the developed extraction technique and analytical method in hair samples. The aforementioned outcomes indicate that the developed and validated HPLC method was successfully applied to hair samples, yet, in the extent of this study only external spiking-based extraction method was tested. Therefore, any matrix effect or loss of extraction evaluation could not be achieved with these preliminary results. A further study with hair samples of recreational users may contribute more to extensively investigate the suitability of this analytical method (Madry, Kraemer, and Baumgartner 2020).

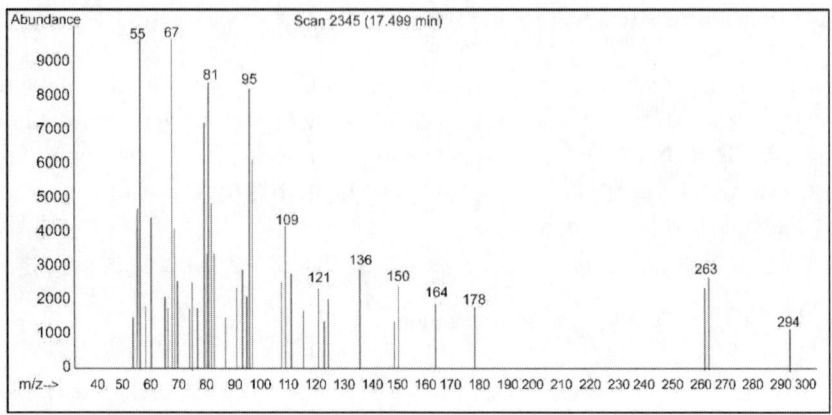

Figure 4. GC-MS spectrum of blank hair sample.

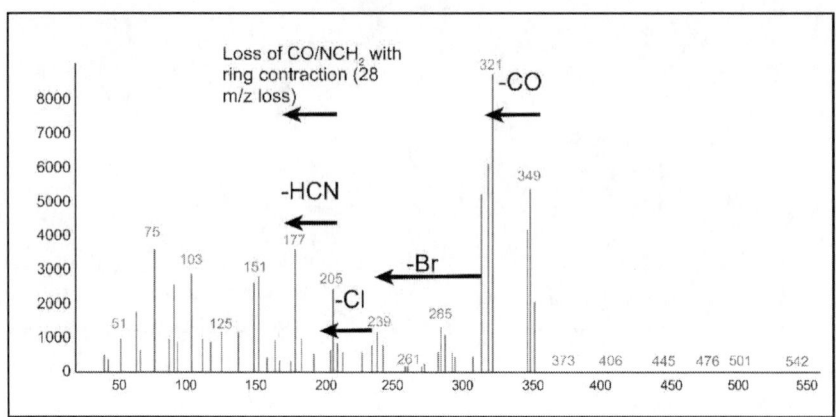

Figure 5. GC-MS result of spiked hair samples matching with phenazepam mass spectrum.

Table 6. Recovery results of spiked hair using optimised method

Concentration (µg/mL)	Measured concentration (µg/mL)	Peak area (mAU x min.)	Mean peak area (mAU x min.)	Recovery %	SD
1000	1000	15.9 18.3 19.1	17.78	100	1.67
100	85	16.3 13.3 15.6	15.07	85	1.57
10	8	13.9 15.2 15.7	14.93	80	0.93

SD: Standard Deviation.

Furthermore, this method should further test for other matrices as well considering phenazepam is commonly encountered in emergency, DIUD, seized drugs, drug facilitated crimes and post-mortem biological samples (McAuley et al., 2015; Bailey et al., 2010; Park et al., 2013; Bollinger et al., 2021; Brunetti et al., 2021; Acikkol, Mercan, and Karadayi 2009). For example, Dargan et al., published a hospitalized case whose serum concentration was found to be 0.49 µg/mL by GC-MS (Dargan et al., 2013). Another study from Finland found phenazepam in several DIUD cases, blood concentrations ranged from 0.022 to 0.85 µg/mL (Heide et al., 2020). With a future well-established extraction procedure for blood, this method could be useful to detect the phenazepam, considering the LOD and LOQ values obtained. On the other hand, when studies in the literature containing phenazepam analysis were examined, a popular technique seems to be LC-MS/MS, due to the sensitivity advantages, with LOD values much lower than this study, revealing the limitation of this work (Crichton et al., 2015; Pettersson Bergstrand, Helander, and Beck 2016). The presumptive detection of NPS-benzodiazepines by immunoassay methods is another possibility, however these techniques are in need of confirmation by advanced chromatographic techniques (Pettersson Bergstrand, Helander, and Beck 2016; Reschly-Krasowski and Krasowski 2018). Therefore, largely MS, electron capture detection or UV detectors coupled to GC or LC systems are required to examine and interpret complex matrices and possible multi-drug content NPS groups. However, considering the affordability and ease of use, HPLC coupled with UV detectors are rather common in clinical and forensic laboratory settings. Hence, it is our belief that this method will be very efficient at points where the aim is mostly clinical and/or forensic detection and quick intervention.

Additionally, 3-hydroxyphenazepam is an active metabolite of phenazepam being sold as a separate NPS-benzodiazepine itself on the market. Some studies identify both from post-mortem samples, yet no correlation was found between them yet (Crichton et al., 2015; Brunetti et al., 2021; EMCDDA 2018). Since the metabolite is also marketed as a recreational drug itself, care must be taken when interpreting. In the future, the proposed method can be extended by adding 3-hydroxyphenazepam and some other NPS-benzodiazepines to achieve a simultaneous investigation, considering the validated method will also be suitable for other 1,4-benzoadiazepines with some minor alterations.

Although NPS-benzodiazepines appear to be only a low percentage of overall NPS seizures (synthetic cannabinoids and cathinones are mostly seized), non-medical use of benzodiazepines is a global threat that cannot be ignored. After World health organization report, United Nations Commission on narcotic drugs added phenazepam to the Schedule IV of the 1971 United Nations convention on psychoactive substances in 2016 (UN CND 2016). The psychoactive substances act was then introduced in the UK for preventing the production of NPS in order to circumvent legislation (UK Home Office 2018). Despite all these legal efforts, phenazepam has still presented itself at intervals in the drug market being one of the most often reported NPS-benzodiazepines along with etizolam and flubromazolam (EMCDDA 2018). Between 2016 and 2019, the most common designer benzodiazepines in forensic cases in Norway were diclazepam and Phenazepam (Heide et al., 2020). In Scotland, there is a large illicit diazepam market, and diazepam is frequently detected with phenazepam, implying that the illicitly made diazepam pills include phenazepam as well (Shearer et al., 2015). Despite all this non-medical use information, it is still not on the controlled drugs' lists of several countries, including Russia, Estonia, Latvia, Lithuania and Belarus, since it is still used as a therapeutic drug that can be prescribed. The United States is another country where phenazepam is not regulated as a controlled substance, despite the fact that many other Benzodiazepines are (DEA 2020).

Conclusion

Although BZD make just a small percentage of the total number of NPS, their use and abuse has grown fast due to its perception as therapeutic substances. In clinical admissions, DUIDs, post-mortem toxicology results, and seizures, phenazepam remains an active ingredient in NPS-benzodiazepines in many countries.

An analytical method validation has been carried out for the clinical and forensic detection of phenazepam and this method was successfully applied to authentic hair samples by externally spiking. Moreover, the validated method also has the potential to be applied in a practical way to seized substances, drug facilitated crimes and clinical intoxications. Hence, the proposed analytical method performed on HPLC- UV/Vis is proven to be a suitable, affordable, and rapid technique for qualitative and quantitative investigation of phenazepam.

Disclaimer

None

Acknowledgments

The authors are thankfully acknowledged Kingston University, London for funding this master's degree study. The corresponding author would like to thank Assoc. Prof. Selda Mercan for her valuable contributions.

References

Acikkol, M., Mercan, S., and Karadayi, S. Simultaneous Determination of Benzodiazepines and Ketamine from Alcoholic and Nonalcoholic Beverages by GC-MS in Drug Facilitated Crimes. *Chromatographia* (2009) 70 (7–8). Friedr. Vieweg und Sohn Verlags GmbH: 1295–1298. doi:10.1365/s10337-009-1278-6.

Bailey, K., Richards-Waugh, L., Clay, D., Gebhardt, M., Mahmoud, H., and Kraner, J. C. Fatality Involving the Ingestion of Phenazepam and Poppy Seed Tea. *Journal of Analytical Toxicology* (2010) 34 (8): 527–532. doi:10.1093/jat/34.8.527.

Belova, M. V., Klyuyev, E. A., Melnikov, E. S., and Yeliseyeva, D. M. Chemical and Toxicological Diagnosis of Acute Poisonings with Phenazepam. *Sklifosovsky Journal Emergency Medical Care* (2018) 7 (4): 319–324. doi:10.23934/2223-9022-2018-7-4-319-324.

Bollinger, K., Weimer, B. L., Heller, D., Bynum, N., Grabenauer, M., Pressley, D. M., and Smiley-McDonald, H. Benzodiazepines Reported in NFLIS-Drug, 2015 to 2018. *Forensic Science International: Synergy 3.* Elsevier Ltd (2021) 100138. doi:10.1016/j.fsisyn. 2021.100138.

Brunetti, P., Giorgetti, R., Tagliabracci, A., Huestis, M. A., and Busardò, F. P. Designer Benzodiazepines: A Review of Toxicology and Public Health Risks. *Pharmaceuticals* (2021) 14 (6): 1–46. doi:10.3390/ph14060560.

Cooper, G. A. A., Kronstrand, R., and Kintz, P. Society of Hair Testing Guidelines for Drug Testing in Hair. *Forensic Science International* (2012) 218 (1–3): 20–24. doi:10.1016/J.FORSCIINT.2011.10.024.

Crichton, M. L., Shenton, C. F., Drummond, G., Beer, L. J., Seetohul, L. N., and Maskell, P. D. Analysis of Phenazepam and 3-Hydroxyphenazepam in Post-Mortem Fluids and Tissues. *Drug Testing and Analysis* (2015) 7 (10): 926–936. doi:10.1002/dta.1790.

Dargan, P. I., Davies, S., Puchnarewicz, M., Johnston, A., and Wood, D. M. First Reported Case in the UK of Acute Prolonged Neuropsychiatric Toxicity Associated with Analytically Confirmed Recreational Use of Phenazepam. *European Journal of Clinical Pharmacology* (2013) 69 (3): 361–363. doi:10.1007/s00228-012-1361-z.

Drug Enforcement Administration (DEA). 2020. *Phenazepam Report.*
European Monitoring Centre for Drugs and Drug Addiction (EMCDDA)-The European Union Agency for Law Enforcement Cooperation (Europol). 2007 Annual Report on the Implementation of Council Decision 2005/387/JHA In Accordance with Article 10 of Council Decision 2005/387/JHA on Information Exchange, Risk Assessment and Control of New Psychoactive Substances. Luxembourg: Publications Office of the European Union, 2007. https://www.emcdda.europa.eu/system/files/publications/503/2007_Implementation_report_281403.pdf.
European Monitoring Centre for Drugs and Drug Addiction (EMCDDA). *The Misuse of Benzodiazepines among High-Risk Opioid Users in Europe.* Perspectives on Drugs. Luxembourg: Publications Office of the European Union, 2018. www.emcdda. europa.eu/publications/manuals/tdi%0Aemcdda.europa.eu/topics/%0Apods/benzodia zepines.
European Monitoring Centre for Drugs and Drug Addiction (EMCDDA). *New Benzodiazepines in Europe – a Review.* Luxembourg: Publications Office of the European Union, 2021. doi:10.2810/725973.
Gerostamoulos, D., Elliott, S., Walls, H. C., Peters, F. T., Lynch, M., and Drummer, O. H. To Measure or Not to Measure? That Is the NPS Question. *Journal of Analytical Toxicology* (2016). doi:10.1093/jat/bkw013.
Heide, G., Høiseth, G., Middelkoop, G., and Øiestad, Å. M. L. Blood Concentrations of Designer Benzodiazepines: Relation to Impairment and Findings in Forensic Cases. *Journal of Analytical Toxicology* (2020) 44 (8): 905–914. doi:10.1093/jat/bkaa043.
International Conference on Harmonization (ICH). M10 Bioanalytical Method Validation. 2019.
Kerrigan, S., Brady-Mellon, M., and Hinners, P. Detection of Phenazepam in Impaired Driving. *Journal of Analytical Toxicology* (2013) 37 (8): 605–610. doi:10.1093/jat/bkt075.
Kriikku, P., Wilhelm, L., Rintatalo, J., Hurme, J., Kramer, J., and Ojanperä, I. Phenazepam Abuse in Finland: Findings from Apprehended Drivers, Post-Mortem Cases and Police Confiscations. *Forensic Science International* (2012) 220 (1–3): 111–117. doi:10. 1016/j.forsciint.2012.02.006.
Lim, W. J. L., Yap, A. T. W., Mangudi, M., Koh, H. B., Tang, A. S. Y., and Chan, K. B. Detection of Phenazepam in Illicitly Manufactured Erimin 5 Tablets. *Drug Testing and Analysis* (2017) 9 (2): 293–305. doi:10.1002/dta.1981.
Madry, M. M., Kraemer, T., and Baumgartner, M. R. Large Scale Consumption Monitoring of Benzodiazepines and Z-Drugs by Hair Analysis. *Journal of Pharmaceutical and Biomedical Analysis* (2020) 183: 113151. doi:10.1016/j.jpba.2020.113151.
Manchester, K. R., Lomas, E. C., Waters, L., Dempsey, F. C., and Maskell, P. D. The Emergence of New Psychoactive Substance (NPS) Benzodiazepines: A Review. *Drug Testing and Analysis* (2018) 10 (1): 37–53. doi:10.1002/dta.2211.
McAuley, A., Hecht, G., Barnsdale, L., Thomson, C. S., Graham, L., Priyadarshi, S., and Robertson, J. R. Mortality Related to Novel Psychoactive Substances in Scotland, 2012: An Exploratory Study. *International Journal of Drug Policy* (2015) 26 (5): 461–467. doi:10.1016/j.drugpo.2014.10.010.

Moosmann, B., and Auwärter, V. Designer Benzodiazepines: Another Class of New Psychoactive Substances. In *Handbook of Experimental Pharmacology* (2018) 252:383–410. doi:10.1007/164_2018_154.

Park, Y., Lee, C., Lee, H., Pyo, J., Jo, J., Lee, J., Choi, H., Kim, S., Hong, R. S., Park, Y., Hwang, B. Y., Choe, S. and Jung, J. H. Identification of a New Synthetic Cannabinoid in a Herbal Mixture: 1-Butyl-3-(2-Methoxybenzoyl)Indole. *Forensic Toxicology* (2013) 31 (2): 187–196. doi:10.1007/s11419-012-0173-2.

Pettersson Bergstrand, M., Helander, A., and Beck, O. Development and Application of a Multi-Component LC–MS/MS Method for Determination of Designer Benzodiazepines in Urine. *Journal of Chromatography B: Analytical Technologies in the Biomedical and Life Sciences* (2016)1035: 104–110. doi:10.1016/j.jchromb.2016.08.047.

Reschly-Krasowski, J. M., and Krasowski, M. D. A Difficult Challenge for the Clinical Laboratory: Accessing and Interpreting Manufacturer Cross-Reactivity Data for Immunoassays Used in Urine Drug Testing. *Academic Pathology* (2018) 5: 237428951881179. doi:10.1177/2374289518811797.

Shearer, K., Bryce, C., Parsons, M., and Torrance, H. Phenazepam: A Review of Medico-Legal Deaths in South Scotland between 2010 and 2014. *Forensic Science International* (2015) 254: 197–204. doi:10.1016/j.forsciint.2015.07.033.

Stephenson, J. B., Golz, D. E., and Brasher, M. J. Phenazepam and Its Effects on Driving. *Journal of Analytical Toxicology* (2013) 37 (1): 25–29. doi:10.1093/jat/bks080.

UK Home Office. *Review of the Psychoactive Substances Act 2016*. 2018. www.gov.uk/government/publications.

UN CND. *UN Commission on Narcotic Drugs*. New York: 2016. http://www.unodc.org/unodc/en/commissions/CND/Subsidiary_Bodies/HONLAC/HONLAC_Index.html.

Vogel, M., Knöpfli, B., Schmid, O., Prica, M., Strasser J, Prieto L, Wiesbeck G A, and Dürsteler-MacFarland K M. Treatment or 'High': Benzodiazepine Use in Patients on Injectable Heroin or Oral Opioids. *Addictive Behaviors* (2013) 38 (10): 2477–2484. doi:10.1016/j.addbeh.2013.05.008.

World Health Organization (WHO). *Phenazepam Pre-Review Report*. Geneva: 2015.

Biographical Sketch

James Barker

Affiliation: Royal Society of Chemistry
The Chartered Society of Forensic Sciences

Education:
1992 PhD: University of Manchester, UK
1988, BSc (Hons) Chemistry: University of Manchester, UK

Business Address: School of Life Sciences, Pharmacy and Chemistry, Kingston University, Penrhyn Road, Kingston-upon-Thames, Surrey, UK, KT1 2EE. Tel: +44 (0) 208 417 2981

Research and Professional Experience
PGCE(HE): University of Greenwich, 1997 and Accredited Teacher in HE: SEDA, 1997
Member of Chartered Society of Forensic Sciences (MCSFS), 2014
Chartered Scientist (CSci): Science Council, 2004
Fellow of Higher Education Academy (FHEA): 2000
European Chemist (EurChem): Eur. Commun. Chem. Council, 1994
Chart'd Chem, Chart'd Science Teacher & Fellow: Royal Society of Chemistry, 1991/2014/2003

Professional Appointments
LSPC School Director of Postgraduate Research
LSPC School Deputy Director of Research and Enterprise
Analytical and Forensic Chemistry Subject Area Leader
Departmental ERASMUS Coordinator

Publications from the Last 3 Years
1. Nassour, Carla, Zacharauskas, Zilvinas, Nabhani-Gebara, Shereen, Barton, Stephen and Barker, James (2022) Development and validation of an ICP-MS method for the detection of platinum in the Lebanese aquatic environment. *Water*, 14(17), p. 2631. ISSN (online) 2073-4441.
2. Salhab, Hassan and Barker, James (2022) Development and validation of an HPLC-UV method for the quantification of 4′-Hydroxydiclofenac using salicylic acid : future applications for measurement of in vitro drug–drug interaction in rat liver microsomes. *Molecules*, 27(11), p. 3587. ISSN (online) 1420-3049.
3. Nassour, Carla, Barker, James, Nabhani-Gebara, Shereen and Barton, Stephen (2022) What's in the water? Shining a light on the impacts of anticancer drugs in our rivers and lakes. *AWE International*, May 2022, pp. 15-23. ISSN (print) 1745-3623.
4. Hussain, Amira, Naughton, Declan P. and Barker, James (2022) Potential effects of ibuprofen, remdesivir and omeprazole on dexamethasone metabolism in control Sprague Dawley male rat liver microsomes (drugs often used together alongside COVID-19 treatment). *Molecules*, 27(7), p. 2238. ISSN (online) 1420-3049.

5. Emamverdian, Abolghassem, Ding, Yulong, Barker, James, Liu, Guohua, Hasanuzzaman, Mirza, Li, Yang, Ramakrishnan, Muthusamy and Mokhberdoran, Farzad (2022) Co-application of 24-epibrassinolide and titanium oxide nanoparticles promotes 'Pleioblastus pygmaeus' plant tolerance to Cu and Cd toxicity by increasing antioxidant activity and photosynthetic capacity and reducing heavy metal accumulation and translocation. *Antioxidants*, 11(3), p. 451. ISSN (online) 2076-3921.
6. Emamverdian, Abolghassem, Hasanuzzaman, Mirza, Ding, Yulong, Barker, James, Mokhberdoran, Farzad and Liu, Guohua (2022) Zinc oxide nanoparticles improve 'Pleioblastus pygmaeus' plant tolerance to arsenic and mercury by stimulating antioxidant defense and reducing the metal accumulation and translocation. *Frontiers in Plant Science*, 13, p. 841501. ISSN (online) 1664-462X.
7. Hussain, Amira, Naughton, Declan P. and Barker, James (2022) Development and validation of a novel HPLC method to analyse metabolic reaction products catalysed by the CYP3A2 isoform : in vitro inhibition of CYP3A2 enzyme activity by aspirin (drugs often used together in COVID-19 treatment). *Molecules*, 27(3), p. 927. ISSN (online) 1420-3049.
8. Taylor, Luke, Saskőy, Lili, Brodie, Tara, Remeškevičius, Vytautas, Moir, Hannah Jayne, Barker, James, Fletcher, John, Thatti, Baljit Kaur, Trotter, Gavin and Rooney, Brian (2022) Development of a gas-tight syringe headspace GC-FID method for the detection of ethanol, and a description of the legal and practical framework for its analysis, in samples of English and Welsh motorists' blood and urine. *Molecules*, 27(15), p. 4771. ISSN (online) 1420-3049.
9. Emamverdian, Abolghassem, Ding, Yulong, Barker, James, Mokhberdoran, Farzad, Ramakrishnan, Muthusamy, Guohua, Liu and Li, Yang (2021) Nitric oxide ameliorates plant tolerance for metal toxicity by increasing antioxidant capacity and reducing heavy metal accumulation and translocation. *Antioxidants*, 10(12), p. 1981. ISSN (online) 2076-3921.
10. Nassour, Carla, Nabhani-Gebara, Shereen, Barton, Stephen J. and Barker, James (2021) Aquatic ecotoxicology of anticancer drugs : a systematic review. *Science of The Total Environment*, 800, p. 149598. ISSN (print) 0048-9697.
11. Mostafa, Aya M., Barton, Stephen J., Wren, Stephen P. and Barker, James (2021) Review on molecularly imprinted polymers with a focus

on their application to the analysis of protein biomarkers. *TrAC Trends in Analytical Chemistry*, 144, p. 116431. ISSN (print) 0165-9936.
12. Cheung, Philip C. W., Williams, Daryl R., Barrett, Jack, Barker, James and Kirk, Donald W. (2021) On the origins of some spectroscopic properties of "purple iron" (the tetraoxoferrate(VI) ion) and its Pourbaix safe-space. *Molecules*, 26(17), p. 5266. ISSN (online) 1420-3049.
13. Salhab, Hassan, Naughton, Declan P. and Barker, James (2021) Potential assessment of UGT2B17 inhibition by salicylic acid in human supersomes in vitro. *Molecules*, 26(15), p. 4410. ISSN (online) 1420-3049.
14. Alhefeiti, Manal A., Barker, James and Shah, Iltaf (2021) Roadside drug testing approaches. *Molecules*, 26(11), p. 3291. ISSN (online) 1420-3049.
15. Langat, Moses K., Mayowa, Yisau, Sadgrove, Nicholas, Danyaal, Mohammed, Prescott, Thomas A. K., Kami, Teva, Schwikkard, Sianne, Barker, James and Cheek, Martin (2021) Multi-layered antimicrobial synergism of (E)-caryophyllene with minor compounds, tecleanatalensine B and normelicopine, from the leaves of 'Vepris gossweileri' (I. Verd.) Mziray. *Natural Product Research*, ISSN (print) 1478-6419 (Epub Ahead of Print).
16. Morrison, Isaac J., Zhang, Jianan, Lin, Jingwen, Murray, JeAnn E., Porter, Roy, Langat, Moses K., Sadgrove, Nicholas J., Barker, James, Zhang, Guodong and Delgoda, Rupika (2021) Potential chemopreventive, anticancer and anti-inflammatory properties of a refined artocarpin-rich wood extract of 'Artocarpus heterophyllus' Lam. *Scientific Reports*, 11, p. 6854. ISSN (online) 2045-2322.
17. Aseperi, Adeniyi K., Busquets, Rosa, Hooda, Peter S., Cheung, Philip C. W. and Barker, James (2020) Behaviour of neonicotinoids in contrasting soils. *Journal of Environmental Management*, 276, p. 111329. ISSN (print) 0301-4797.
18. Patel, Rahul, Barker, James and Elshaer, Amr (2020) Pharmaceutical excipients and drug metabolism : a mini-review. *International journal of molecular sciences*, 21(21), p. 8224. ISSN (online) 1422-0067.
19. Adegun, Ayodeji O., Akinnifesi, Thompson A., Ololade, Isaac A., Busquets, Rosa, Hooda, Peter S., Cheung, Philip C. W., Aseperi, Adeniyi K. and Barker, James (2020) Quantification of neonicotinoid pesticides in six cultivable fish species from the River Owena in Nigeria and a template for food safety assessment. *Water*, 12(9), p. 2422. ISSN (online) 2073-4441.

20. Ibrahim, Ghada Rashad, Shah, Iltaf, Gariballa, Salah, Yasin, Javed, Barker, James and Ashraf, Syed Salman (2020) Significantly elevated levels of plasma nicotinamide, pyridoxal, and pyridoxamine phosphate levels in obese Emirati population : a cross-sectional study. *Molecules*, 25(17), p. 3932. ISSN (online) 1420-3049.
21. Meissner, Wlodzimierz, Binkowski, Lukasz J., Barker, James, Hahn, Andreas and Trzeciak, Marta (2020) Relationship between blood lead levels and physiological stress in mute swans ('Cygnus olor') in municipal beaches of the southern Baltic. *Science of the Total Environment*, 710, p. 136292. ISSN (print) 0048-9697.
22. Salhab, Hassan, Naughton, Declan P. and Barker, James (2020) Validation of an HPLC method for the simultaneous quantification of metabolic reaction products catalysed by CYP2E1 enzyme activity : inhibitory effect of cytochrome P450 enzyme CYP2E1 by salicylic acid in rat liver microsomes. *Molecules*, 25(4), p. 932. ISSN (online) 1420-3049.
23. Nassour, Carla, Barton, Stephen J., Nabhani-Gebara, Shereen, Saab, Yolande and Barker, James (2020) Occurrence of anticancer drugs in the aquatic environment : a systematic review. *Environmental Science and Pollution Research*, 27, pp. 1339-1347. ISSN (print) 0944-1344.
24. Foster, Kimberley, Oyenihi, Omolola, Rademan, Sunelle, Erhabor, Joseph, Matsabisa, Motlalepula, Barker, James, Langat, Moses K., Kendal-Smith, Amy, Asemota, Helen and Delgoda, Rupika (2020) Selective cytotoxic and anti-metastatic activity in DU-145 prostate cancer cells induced by 'Annona muricata' L. bark extract and phytochemical, annonacin. *BMC Complementary Medicine and Therapies*, 20, p. 375. ISSN (online) 2662-7671.

Bibliography

Addiction treatment homework planner
LCCN	2013038895
Type of material	Book
Personal name	Finley, James R., 1948- author.
Main title	Addiction treatment homework planner / James R. Finley and Brenda S. Lenz.
Edition	Fifth edition.
Published/Produced	Hoboken, New Jersey: John Wiley and Sons, Inc., [2014]
Description	xviii, 389 pages; 28 cm + 1 CD-ROM (4 3/4 in.)
Links	Cover image http://catalogimages.wiley.com/images/db/jimages/9781118560594.jpg
	Contributor biographical information https://www.loc.gov/catdir/enhancements/fy1702/2013038895-b.html
	Publisher description https://www.loc.gov/catdir/enhancements/fy1702/2013038895-d.html
	Table of contents only https://www.loc.gov/catdir/enhancements/fy1702/2013038895-t.html
ISBN	9781118560594 (pbk.)
	9781119278047
LC classification	RC564.15 .F555 2014
Related names	Lenz, Brenda S., author.
Summary	"The Addiction Treatment Homework Planner provides an array of ready-to-use, between-session assignments designed to fit virtually every treatment setting and therapeutic mode including individual therapy, family therapy, and group counseling. This easy-to-use sourcebook features: 100 ready-to-copy exercises covering the most common issues encountered by clients suffering from chemical and nonchemical addictions, such as anxiety, impulsivity, occupational problems, and childhood problems A quick-reference format - the interactive assignments

	are grouped by behavioral problems including alcoholism, nicotine dependence, and substance abuse, as well as those problems that do not involve psychoactive substances, such as problem gambling, eating disorders, and sexual addictions Offers special attention to the patient placement Criteria (PPC) developed by the American Society of Addiction Medicine (ASAM). A checklist included in the Appendix helps evaluate clients on each of the ASAM six assessment dimensions Expert guidance on how and when to make the most efficient use of the exercises A CD-ROM that contains all the exercises allows you to customize the exercises to suit you and your clients' unique styles and needs "-- Provided by publisher.
LC Subjects	Substance abuse--Treatment--Handbooks, manuals, etc.
	Substance abuse--Treatment--Planning.
Other Subjects	Psychology / Psychopathology / Addiction.
Notes	Includes bibliographical references.
Additional formats	Online version: Finley, James R., 1948- author. Addiction treatment homework planner Fifth edition. Hoboken, New Jersey: John Wiley and Sons, Inc., [2014] 9781118836514 (DLC) 2013039176
Series	PracticePlanners series

Addiction treatment homework planner

LCCN	2013039176
Type of material	Book
Personal name	Finley, James R., 1948- author.
Main title	Addiction treatment homework planner / James R. Finley and Brenda S. Lenz.
Edition	Fifth edition.
Published/Produced	Hoboken, New Jersey: John Wiley and Sons, Inc., [2014]
Description	1 online resource.
Links	Cover image http://catalogimages.wiley.com/images/db/jimages/9781118560594.jpg
ISBN	9781118836279 (epub)

	9781118836514 (pdf)
LC classification	RC564.15
Related names	Lenz, Brenda S., author.
Summary	"The Addiction Treatment Homework Planner provides an array of ready-to-use, between-session assignments designed to fit virtually every treatment setting and therapeutic mode including individual therapy, family therapy, and group counseling. This easy-to-use sourcebook features: 100 ready-to-copy exercises covering the most common issues encountered by clients suffering from chemical and nonchemical addictions, such as anxiety, impulsivity, occupational problems, and childhood problems A quick-reference format - the interactive assignments are grouped by behavioral problems including alcoholism, nicotine dependence, and substance abuse, as well as those problems that do not involve psychoactive substances, such as problem gambling, eating disorders, and sexual addictions Offers special attention to the patient placement Criteria (PPC) developed by the American Society of Addiction Medicine (ASAM). A checklist included in the Appendix helps evaluate clients on each of the ASAM six assessment dimensions Expert guidance on how and when to make the most efficient use of the exercises A CD-ROM that contains all the exercises allows you to customize the exercises to suit you and your clients' unique styles and needs "-- Provided by publisher.
LC Subjects	Substance abuse--Treatment--Handbooks, manuals, etc.
	Substance abuse--Treatment--Planning.
Other Subjects	Psychology / Psychopathology / Addiction.
Notes	Includes bibliographical references.
Additional formats	Print version: Finley, James R., 1948- author. Addiction treatment homework planner Fifth edition. Hoboken, New Jersey: John Wiley and Sons, Inc., [2014] 9781118560594 (DLC) 2013038895
Series	Practice Planners series

Addictive substances and neurological disease: alcohol, tobacco, caffeine, and drugs of abuse in everyday lifestyles

LCCN	2016960662
Type of material	Book
Main title	Addictive substances and neurological disease: alcohol, tobacco, caffeine, and drugs of abuse in everyday lifestyles / edited by Ronald Ross Watson, University of Arizona, Arizona Health Sciences Center, Tucson, AZ, USA, Sherma Zibadi, Department of Pathology, University of South Florida Medical School, Tampa, FL, USA.
Published/Produced	London, United Kingdom; San Diego, CA, United States: Elsevier/AP, Academic Press, an imprint of Elsevier [2017]
Description	xv, 398 pages: illustrations (chiefly color); 29 cm
ISBN	9780128053737 (hardcover)
	0128053739 (hardcover)
LC classification	RC564.A3265 2017
Related names	Watson, Ronald R. (Ronald Ross), editor.
	Zibadi, Sherma, editor.
Summary	Addictive Substances and Neurological Disease: Alcohol, Tobacco, Caffeine, and Drugs of Abuse in Everyday Lifestyles is a complete guide to the manifold effects of addictive substances on the brain, providing readers with the latest developing research on how these substances are implicated in neurological development and dysfunction. Cannabis, cocaine, and other illicit drugs can have substantial negative effects on the structure and functioning of the brain. However, other common habituating and addictive substances often used as part of an individual's lifestyle, i.e., alcohol, tobacco, caffeine, painkillers can also compromise brain health and effect or accentuate neurological disease. This book provides broad coverage of the effects of addictive substances on the brain, beginning with an overview of how the substances lead to dysfunction before examining each substance in depth. It discusses the pathology of addiction, the structural

Contents

damage resulting from abuse of various substances, and covers the neurobiological, neurodegenerative, behavioral, and cognitive implications of use across the lifespan, from prenatal exposure, to adolescence and old age. This book aids researchers seeking an understanding of the neurological changes that these substances induce, and is also extremely useful for those seeking potential treatments and therapies for individuals suffering from chronic abuse of these substances.-- Source other than Library of Congress. Acute ethanol-induced changes in microstructural and metabolite concentrations on the brain: noninvasive functional brain Imaging - Prenatal alcohol exposure and neuroglial changes in neurochemistry and behavior in animal models - Alcohol on histaminergic neurons of brain - Antenatal alcohol and histological brain disturbances - Alcohol intoxication and traumatic spinal cord injury: basic and clinical science - Visual and auditory changes after acute alcohol ingestion - Zebrafish models of alcohol addiction - Effect of alcohol on the regulation of a-Synnuclein in the human brain - Consumption of ethanol and tissue changes in the central nervous system - Ethanol consumption and cerebellar disorders - Gene expression in CNS regions of genetic rat models of alcohol abuse - Role of TLR4 in the ethanol-induced modulation of the autophagy pathway in the brain - Ghrelinergic signaling in ethanol reward - Alcoholic neurological syndromes - Frontal lobe dysfunction after developmental alcohol exposure: implications from animal models - Ethanol's action mechanisms in the brain: from lipid general alterations to specific protein receptor binding - Antioxidant vitamins and brain dysfunction in alcoholics - Serotonin deficiency and alcohol use disorders - Functional reorganization of reward- and habit-related brain networks in addiction - Ethanol: neurotoxicity and brain disorders - Functionally relevant brain alterations in

	polysubstance users: differences to monosubstance users, study challenges, and implications for treatment - Deep brain stimulation: a possible therapeutic technique for treating refractory alcohol and drug addiction behaviors - Understanding the roles of genetic and environmental influences on the neurobiology of nicotine use - Tobacco smoke and nicotine: neurotoxicity in brain development - Paradise lost: a new paradigm for explaining the interaction between neural and psychological changes in nicotine addiction patients - Interactions of alcohol and nicotine: CNS sites and contributions to their co-abuse - Role of basal forebrain in nicotine alcohol co-abuse - Chronic and acute nicotine exposure versus placebo in smokers and nonsmokers: a systematic review of resting-state fMRI studies - Novel psychoactive substances: a new behavioral and mental health threat - Cholesterol and caffeine modulate alcohol actions on cerebral arteries and brain - Sleep, caffeine, and physical activity in older adults - Ketamine: neurotoxicity and neurobehavioral disorders - Left/right hemispheric "unbalance" model in addiction.
LC Subjects	Substance abuse--Physiological aspects. Substance abuse--Psychological aspects. Drugs of abuse--Physiological effect. Nervous system--Diseases.
Other Subjects	Substance-Related Disorders--complications. Neurologic Manifestations. Behavior, Addictive--physiopathology. Drugs of abuse--Physiological effect. Nervous system--Diseases. Substance abuse--Physiological aspects. Substance abuse--Psychological aspects.
Notes	Includes bibliographical references and index.

ADHD is not an illness and ritalin is not a cure: a comprehensive rebuttal of the (alleged) scientific consensus

LCCN	2022004980

Bibliography

Type of material	Book
Personal name	Ophir, Yaakov, author.
Main title	ADHD is not an illness and ritalin is not a cure: a comprehensive rebuttal of the (alleged) scientific consensus / Yaakov Ophir, Technion - Israel Institute of Technology, Israel.
Published/Produced	Hackensack, NJ: World Scientific, [2022]
ISBN	9789811253225 (hardcover)
	9789811254130 (paperback)
	(ebook for institutions)
	(ebook for individuals)
LC classification	RJ506.H9 O64 2022
Summary	"Is Attention Deficit Hyperactivity Disorder (ADHD), the most prevalent neuropsychiatric label in children, a valid medical condition? Should we really refer to the millions of children diagnosed with ADHD as children who suffer from the "diabetes of psychiatry" - a chronic and harmful biological condition that must be treated regularly with powerful psychoactive substances? Building on previous critiques, this thorough, elegant, and mainly courageous book answers these questions through a step-by-step rebuttal of the scientific consensus about ADHD and its first-line treatment with stimulant medications. Although the book consists of high-resolution inspection of methodologies, research findings, and writing tactics, it is written in a clear, creative, and flowing way, using colorful examples - some funny, some tragic - which sweep the reader and inspire a societal change. Essentially, the book integrates key critiques into one consolidated source, uncovers the massive evidence against the efficacy and safety of stimulant medications, and provides future directions for socio-educational/parental solutions to this burning public-health problem. But most importantly, this book reviews dozens of dozens of reliability and validity gaps in the overriding (and somewhat aggressive) bio-medical consensus. In this way, the book serves as the missing needle that is

	required to finally pierce the over-blown, and already full of holes theoretical balloon, known as ADHD"-- Provided by publisher.
LC Subjects	Attention-deficit hyperactivity disorder.
	Methylphenidate.
Notes	Includes bibliographical references and index.

Adolescent co-occurring substance use and mental health disorders

LCCN	2022010873
Type of material	Book
Main title	Adolescent co-occurring substance use and mental health disorders / Ken C. Winters and Ann Ingwalson.
Published/Produced	New York, NY: Oxford University Press, [2022]
ISBN	9780190678487 (hardback)
	(epub)
LC classification	RJ506.D78 A358 2022
Related names	Winters, Ken C., editor.
	Ingwalson, Ann, editor.
Contents	Physical and psychosocial development - Adolescent brain development - Overview of psychoactive substances - Substance use disorders - Internalizing and related disorders - Externalizing and related disorders - Process addictions - Continuum of care and treatment planning - Cognitive behavior and dialectic behavior therapies - Motivational enhancement treatment - Family-based treatments - 12-step-based-treatment.
LC Subjects	Teenagers--Substance use.
	Substance abuse--Treatment.
	Teenagers--Mental health.
	Teenagers--Mental health services.
	Comorbidity.
Notes	Includes bibliographical references and index.
Additional formats	Online version: Adolescent co-occurring substance use and mental health disorders New York, NY: Oxford University Press, [2022] 9780190678500 (DLC) 2022010874

Adolescent co-occurring substance use and mental health disorders
LCCN	2022010874
Type of material	Book
Main title	Adolescent co-occurring substance use and mental health disorders / Ken C. Winters and Ann Ingwalson.
Published/Produced	New York, NY: Oxford University Press, [2022]
Description	1 online resource
ISBN	9780190678517
	9780190678500 (epub)
	(hardback)
LC classification	RJ506.D78
Related names	Winters, Ken C., editor.
	Ingwalson, Ann, editor.
Contents	Physical and psychosocial development - Adolescent brain development - Overview of psychoactive substances - Substance use disorders - Internalizing and related disorders - Externalizing and related disorders - Process addictions - Continuum of care and treatment planning - Cognitive behavior and dialectic behavior therapies - Motivational enhancement treatment - Family-based treatments - 12-step-based-treatment.
LC Subjects	Teenagers--Substance use.
	Substance abuse--Treatment.
	Teenagers--Mental health.
	Teenagers--Mental health services.
	Comorbidity.
Notes	Includes bibliographical references and index.
Additional formats	Print version: Adolescent co-occurring substance use and mental health disorders New York, NY: Oxford University Press, [2022] 9780190678487 (DLC) 2022010873

Advances in Intelligent Data Analysis XV: 15th International Symposium, IDA 2016, Stockholm, Sweden, October 13-15, 2016, Proceedings
LCCN	2019761653
Type of material	Book

Main title	Advances in Intelligent Data Analysis XV: 15th International Symposium, IDA 2016, Stockholm, Sweden, October 13-15, 2016, Proceedings / edited by Henrik Boström, Arno Knobbe, Carlos Soares, Panagiotis Papapetrou.
Edition	1st ed. 2016.
Published/Produced	Cham: Springer International Publishing: Imprint: Springer, 2016.
Description	1 online resource (XIII, 404 pages 146 illustrations) PDF
ISBN	9783319463490
Related names	Boström, Henrik. editor. Knobbe, Arno. editor. Papapetrou, Panagiotis. editor. Soares, Carlos. editor.
Summary	This book constitutes the refereed conference proceedings of the 15th International Conference on Intelligent Data Analysis, which was held in October 2016 in Stockholm, Sweden. The 36 revised full papers presented were carefully reviewed and selected from 75 submissions. The traditional focus of the IDA symposium series is on end-to-end intelligent support for data analysis. The symposium aims to provide a forum for inspiring research contributions that might be considered preliminary in other leading conferences and journals, but that have a potentially dramatic impact.
Contents	DSCo-NG: A Practical Language Modeling Approach for Time Series Classification - Ranking Accuracy for Logistic-GEE models - The Morality Machine: Tracking Moral Values in Tweets - A Hybrid Approach for Probabilistic Relational Models Structure Learning - On the Impact of Data Set Size in Transfer Learning Using Deep Neural Networks - Obtaining Shape Descriptors from a Concave Hull-Based Clustering Algorithm - Visual Perception of Discriminative Landmarks in Classified Time Series - Spotting the Diffusion of New Psychoactive Substances over the Internet - Feature Selection

Issues in Long-Term Travel Time Prediction - A Mean-Field Variational Bayesian Approach to Detecting Overlapping Communities with Inner Roles Using Poisson Link Generation - Online Semi-supervised Learning for Multi-target Regression in Data streams Using AMRules - A Toolkit for Analysis of Deep Learning Experiments - The Optimistic Method for Model Estimation - Does Feature Selection Improve Classification? A Large Scale Experiment in OpenML - Learning from the News: Predicting Entity Popularity on Twitter - Multi-scale Kernel PCA and Its Application to Curvelet-based Feature Extraction for Mammographic Mass Characterization - Weakly-supervised Symptom Recognition for Rare Diseases in Biomedical Text - Estimating Sequence Similarity from Read Sets for Clustering Sequencing Data - Widened Learning of Bayesian Network Classifiers - Vote Buying Detection via Independent Component Analysis - Unsupervised Relation Extraction in Specialized Corpora Using Sequence Mining - A Framework for Interpolating Scattered Data Using Space-filling Curves - Privacy-Awareness of Distributed Data Clustering Algorithms Revisited - Bi-stochastic Matrix Approximation Framework for Data Co-clustering - Sequential Cost-Sensitive Feature Acquisition - Explainable and Efficient Link Prediction in Real-World Network Data - DGRMiner: Anomaly Detection and Explanation in Dynamic Graphs - Similarity Based Hierarchical Clustering with an Application to Text Collections - Determining Data Relevance Using Semantic Types and Graphical Interpretation Cues - A First Step Toward Quantifying the Climate's Information Production over the Last 68,000 Years - HAUCA Curves for the Evaluation of Biomarker Pilot Studies with Small Sample Sizes and Large Numbers of Features - Stability Evaluation of Event Detection Techniques for Twitter - IDA 2016 Industrial

	Challenge: Using Machine Learning for Predicting Failures - An Optimized k-NN Approach for Classification on Imbalanced Datasets with Missing Data - Combining Boosted Trees with Metafeature Engineering for Predictive Maintenance - Prediction of Failures in the Air Pressure System of Scania Trucks Using a Random Forest and Feature Engineering.
LC Subjects	Algorithms. Application software. Artificial intelligence. Data mining. Database management. Information storage and retrieval.
Other Subjects	Database Management. Algorithm Analysis and Problem Complexity. Artificial Intelligence. Data Mining and Knowledge Discovery. Information Storage and Retrieval. Information Systems Applications (incl. Internet).
Additional formats	Print version: Advances in intelligent data analysis. 9783319463483 (DLC) 2016950907 Printed edition: 9783319463483 Printed edition: 9783319463506
Series	Information Systems and Applications, incl. Internet/Web, and HCI; 9897 Information Systems and Applications, incl. Internet/Web, and HCI; 9897

Aggression as a challenge: theory and research: current problems

LCCN	2014047464
Type of material	Book
Main title	Aggression as a challenge: theory and research: current problems / Hanna Liberska, Marzanna Farnicka (eds.).
Edition	1 Edition.
Published/Produced	New York: Peter Lang, edition, [2016]
Description	274 pages; 22 cm
ISBN	9783631656884 (Print: alk. paper)

LC classification	BF575.A3 .A514 2016
Related names	Liberska, Hanna, editor.
	Farnicka, Marzanna, 1974- editor.
Contents	Aggression as a challenge: introduction - Aggression: theoretical issues - Stages and paths of aggression development: the knowledge that awaits being uncovered / M. Farnicka, H. Liberska - Patterns of readiness for interpersonal aggression / A. Fraczek, K. Konopka, K. Dominiak-Kochanek - Aggression the world of children and adolescents - Students' aggressive behaviour at school Czech and Polish comparison / S. Musilova, J. Trempala - Assuming the role of an aggressor and victim by lower secondary school youth: research report / H. Liberska, K. Boniecka, P. Tumendemberel - Peer sexual abuse. phenomenon diagnosis: perpetrators and their therapy / Z. Izdebski, K. Waz - Cyberbullying: the need for prevention in schools / B. Aouil, M. Kajdasz-Aouil, Malgorzata Suprynowicz - Family correlates of adolescents' readiness to assume the role of aggressor or victim / M. Farnicka, I. Grzegorzewska - Anger and attachment of growing up children in biological and foster families / K. Mickiewicz, K. Glogowska - Which aspects of aggression appear due to coping with stress? / A. Kozlowska - Specific risk behaviors and methods for dealing with stress based in religion in teenagers using psychoactive substances / N. Mataczynska, M. Tudorowska - Family dysfuncionality as a risk factor for mood disorders in adolescent / E. Turska - Aggression: a world of adults - Emotional dysregulation and aggression among people with borderline personality disorders / L. Cierpialkowska - Aversive parenting / L. Bakiera - Family determinants and susceptibility of an individual to mobbing at workplace / K. Walczak, K. Walecka-Matyja - Manifestations of aggression in prisoners and their selected determinants / H. Liberska - The level of emotional intelligence among prisoners /

	Boruc - Professional approach and the first line of institutional response of violence against family members (a hungarian overview) / L. Huse, N. Borcz, M. Fonay.
LC Subjects	Aggressiveness.
	Violence.

Analytical methods for environmental contaminants of emerging concern

LCCN	2022012511
Type of material	Book
Main title	Analytical methods for environmental contaminants of emerging concern / edited by Núria Fontanals, Rosa Maria Marcé.
Edition	First edition
Published/Produced	Hoboken, NJ, USA: John Wiley & Sons, 2022.
Description	1 online resource
ISBN	9781119763895 (ebook)
	9781119763871 (pdf)
	9781119763888 (epub)
	(hardback)
LC classification	TD193
Related names	Fontanals, Núria, editor.
	Marcé, Rosa Maria, editor.
Summary	"Provides the analytical methodology required to detect different families of organic compounds of emerging concern (CECs) from environmental samples. Most contaminants of emerging concern (CECs)--such as pharmaceuticals, personal care products, pesticides, sunscreens, perfluorinated compounds, and microplastics--have been present in the environment for years, yet some have only recently been identified, and many of these organic compounds remain unregulated. Analytical methods have been developed to determine the toxicity and risk of different families of CECs. Analytical Methods for Environmental Contaminants of Emerging Concern presents the methods currently available to determine families of organic CECs in

environmental samples. Each section of the book is devoted to a particular family of CECs, covering different analytical methods supported by examples of both cutting-edge research and commonly used methods. An international panel of experts describes every step of the analytical procedures, including sample preparation, chromatographic separation coupled to mass spectrometry or other instrumental techniques. Specific requirements are linked to the properties of the contaminants and the sample matrix for each procedure presented. Throughout the book, in-depth case studies of analytical procedures for CEC extraction, separation, and determination are presented to help readers transfer the analytical methods to their laboratories."

Contents 1. Pesticides - 2. Pharmaceuticals - 3. Personal care products - 4. Novel psychoactive substances - 5. Artificial sweeteners - 6. Perfluorinated substances - 7. High production volume chemicals - 8. Musk fragrances - 9. Disinfection byproducts in water - 10. Microplastics.

LC Subjects Environmental toxicology.
Pollutants--Environmental aspects.
Pollutants--Analysis.

Notes Includes bibliographical references and index.

Additional formats Also available online.
Print version: Analytical methods for environmental contaminants of emerging concern First edition Hoboken, NJ, USA: John Wiley & Sons, 2022 9781119763864 (DLC) 2022012510

Analytical methods for environmental contaminants of emerging concern

LCCN 2022012510
Type of material Book
Main title Analytical methods for environmental contaminants of emerging concern / edited by Núria Fontanals, Rosa Maria Marcé.
Edition First edition

Published/Produced	Hoboken, NJ, USA: John Wiley & Sons, 2022.
ISBN	9781119763864 (hardback)
	(pdf)
	(epub)
	(ebook)
LC classification	TD193.A625 2022
Related names	Fontanals, Núria, editor.
	Marcé, Rosa Maria, editor.
Summary	"Provides the analytical methodology required to detect different families of organic compounds of emerging concern (CECs) from environmental samples. Most contaminants of emerging concern (CECs)--such as pharmaceuticals, personal care products, pesticides, sunscreens, perfluorinated compounds, and microplastics--have been present in the environment for years, yet some have only recently been identified, and many of these organic compounds remain unregulated. Analytical methods have been developed to determine the toxicity and risk of different families of CECs. Analytical Methods for Environmental Contaminants of Emerging Concern presents the methods currently available to determine families of organic CECs in environmental samples. Each section of the book is devoted to a particular family of CECs, covering different analytical methods supported by examples of both cutting-edge research and commonly used methods. An international panel of experts describes every step of the analytical procedures, including sample preparation, chromatographic separation coupled to mass spectrometry or other instrumental techniques. Specific requirements are linked to the properties of the contaminants and the sample matrix for each procedure presented. Throughout the book, in-depth case studies of analytical procedures for CEC extraction, separation, and determination are presented to help readers transfer the analytical methods to their laboratories."

Contents	1. Pesticides - 2. Pharmaceuticals - 3. Personal care products - 4. Novel psychoactive substances - 5. Artificial sweeteners - 6. Perfluorinated substances - 7. High production volume chemicals - 8. Musk fragrances - 9. Disinfection byproducts in water - 10. Microplastics.
LC Subjects	Environmental toxicology. Pollutants--Environmental aspects. Pollutants--Analysis.
Notes	Includes bibliographical references and index.
Additional formats	Also available online. Online version: Analytical methods for environmental contaminants of emerging concern First edition Hoboken, NJ, USA: John Wiley & Sons, 2022 9781119763871 (DLC) 2022012511

Ancient psychoactive substances

LCCN	2017032192
Type of material	Book
Main title	Ancient psychoactive substances / edited by Scott M. Fitzpatrick.
Published/Produced	Gainesville: University Press of Florida, [2018]
Description	ix, 328 pages: illustrations, maps; 24 cm
ISBN	9780813056708 (cloth: acid-free paper)
LC classification	RM315 .A58 2018
Related names	Fitzpatrick, Scott M., editor.
Summary	This book details the traditional and sacred use of psychoactive substances by peoples in the ancient past through the lens of archaeology.
LC Subjects	Psychotropic drugs--History. Hallucinogenic drugs--History. Altered states of consciousness--History. Hallucinogenic drugs and religious experience--History. Drug abuse--History. Alcoholism--History.
Notes	Includes bibliographical references and index.

Chemical health threats: assessing and alerting

LCCN	2019461149
Type of material	Book
Main title	Chemical health threats: assessing and alerting / edited by Raquel Duarte-Davidson, Public Health England, UK, email: Raquel.Durate-Davidson@PHE.gov.uk, Tom Gaulton, Public Health England, UK, email: tom.gaulton@phe.gov.uk, Stacey Wyke, Public Health England, UK, email: Stacey.wyke@phe.gov.uk, and Samuel Collins, Public Health England, UK, email: Samuel.Collins@phe.gov.uk.
Published/Produced	Croydon [England]: The Royal Society of Chemistry, [2019]
Description	xix, 309 pages: color illustrations; 24 cm.
ISBN	9781782620716 (print)
	(pdf)
	(epub)
LC classification	T55.3.H3 C4832 2019
Related names	Duarte-Davidson, Raquel, editor.
	Gaulton, Tom, editor.
	Wyke, Stacey, editor.
	Collins, Samuel (Public health scientist), editor.
Contents	Overview of Alerting, Assessing and Responding to Chemical Public Health Threats / S. Wyke and R. Duarte-Davidson - Chemical Regulation at the European Level: Safeguarding Consumer Health and Protecting the Environment / Ehi Idahoa-Taylor and Samuel Collins - Medical Management of Mass Intoxications / Herbert Desel and Nina Glaser - Hazardous Exposures to Liquid Laundry Detergents Capsules in Young Children / L. Settimi, E. Idahosa-Taylor, S. Wyke and F. Davanzo - Novel Applications of Spatial Mapping to Chemicals or Biological Outbreaks / Paolo Massimo Buscema and Francesca Della Torre - Surveillance of Chemical Health Threats / Tom Gaulton, Rob Orford, Charlotte Hague, Eirian Thomas, and Raquel Duarte-Davidson - Responding to New Psychoactive Substances in the European Union: Early Warning, Risk Assessment

	and Control Measures / M. Evans-Brown, A. Almeida, A. Gallegos, R. Christie, R. Jorge, H. V. Danielsson, T. le Ruez and R. Sedefov - Rapid Public Health Risk Assessments for Emerging Chemical Health Threats / Emma-Jane Goode, Samuel Collins, Charlotte Hague, Rob Orford and Raquel Duarte-Davidson - Review of Risk Management Measures to Mitigate Against Exposures to Household Chemical Consumer Products / S. Wyke and H. Desel - Understanding and Managing Behavioural and Psychological Responses to Chemical Incidents / Richard Amlôt and Holly Carter - Strategic, Technical and Scientific Advice in an Environmental Emergency / Henrietta Harrison and Naima Bradley - Public Health Preparation and Response to Chemical Incident Emergencies / Mark Griffiths - Chemical Incident Management: An Overview of Preparedness, Response and Recovery / Emma Goode, Tom James and Stacey Wyke - Investigating Outbreaks of Unknown Aetiology / S. Collins, T. Gaulton and T. James.
LC Subjects	Hazardous substances--Safety measures--International cooperation.
	Hazardous substances--Health aspects--Europe.
	Hazardous substances--Risk assessment--Europe.
	Hazardous substances--Safety regulations--Europe.
	Hazardous substances--Government policy--Europe.
Notes	Includes bibliographical references and index.
Series	Issues in toxicology; 38

Clinical textbook of addictive disorders

LCCN	2015037303
Type of material	Book
Main title	Clinical textbook of addictive disorders / edited by Avram H. Mack [and three others].
Edition	Fourth edition.
Published/Produced	New York: The Guilford Press, [2016] ©2016
Description	xix, 730 pages: illustrations; 26 cm

ISBN	9781462521692 (hardcover)
	146252169X (hardcover)
	9781462521685 (paperback)
	1462521681 (paperback)
LC classification	RC564 .C55 2016
Related names	Mack, Avram H., editor.
Summary	"This state-of-the-science reference and text has given thousands of practitioners and students a strong foundation in understanding and treating addictive disorders. Leading experts address the neurobiology of addictions and review best practices in assessment and diagnosis. Specific substances of abuse are examined in detail, with attention to real-world clinical considerations. Issues in working with particular populations--including polysubstance abusers, culturally diverse patients, older adults, chronic pain sufferers, and others--are explored. Chapters summarize the theoretical and empirical underpinnings of widely used psychosocial and pharmacological treatments and clearly describe clinical techniques. New to This Edition *Incorporates a decades worth of major advances in research and clinical practice. *Updated for DSM-5. Many new authors; extensively revised with the latest information on specific biological mechanisms, substances, populations, and treatments. *Chapter on motivational interviewing"-- Provided by publisher.
	"This state-of-the-science reference and text has given thousands of practitioners and students a strong foundation in understanding and treating addictive disorders. Leading experts address the neurobiology of addictions and review best practices in assessment and diagnosis. Specific substances of abuse are examined in detail, with attention to real-world clinical considerations. Issues in working with particular populations--including polysubstance abusers, culturally diverse patients, older adults, chronic pain sufferers, and others--are explored. Chapters summarize the theoretical and empirical

underpinnings of widely used psychosocial and pharmacological treatments and clearly describe clinical techniques. Subject Areas/Key Words: addiction medicine, addiction psychiatry, addictions, addictive disorders, adolescents, alcoholism, approaches, assessments, behavioral addictions, biological, dependence, diagnosis, drugs, DSM-5, DSM-V, elderly, evidence-based treatments, gender, geriatric, individualized, interventions, matching, psychopharmacology, substance abuse, substance use disorders, therapy, treatment, women Audience: Psychiatrists, clinical psychologists, social workers, substance abuse and mental health counselors, and psychiatric nurses; graduate students and residents"-- Provided by publisher.

Contents I. Foundations of Addiction - 1. Neurobiology of Substance Use Disorders: Implications for Treatment, Thomas R. Kosten & Colin N. Haile - 2. Historical and Social Context of Psychoactive Substance Disorders, Joseph Westermeyer - II. Assessment of Addiction - 3. Diagnostic Assessment of Substance Abusers, Deborah Hasin & Bari Kilcoyne - 4. Laboratory Testing for Substances of Abuse, D. Andrew Baron & David A. Baron - III. Substances of Abuse - 5. Alcohol, Ed Nace - 6. Nicotine Dependence, David Kalman, Amy Harrington, Joseph DiFranza, Lori Pbert, & Douglas Ziedonis - 7. Opioids, Sudie E. Back, Jenna L. McCauley, Kelly S. Barth, & Kathleen T. Brady - 8. Cannabis, Alicia R. Murray & Frances R. Levin - 9. Hallucinogens and Inhalants, Stephen Ross & Avram H. Mack - 10. Caffeine, Laura M. Juliano & Greta Bielacyzc Raglan - 11. Stimulants, Richard Rawson, Larissa Mooney, & Walter Ling - 12. Cocaine, Evaristo Akerele & Niru Nahar - 13. Sedatives/Hypnotics and Benzodiazepines, Robert L. DuPont, William M. Greene, & Caroline M. DuPont - IV. Special Populations - 14. Polysubstance Use, Abuse, and Dependence, Richard N. Rosenthal,

Petros Levounis, & Abigail J. Herron - 15. Co-Occurring Substance Use Disorders and Other Psychiatric Disorders, Benjamin C. Silverman, Lisa M. Najavits, Roger D. Weiss - 16. Gambling Disorder and Other "Behavioral" Addictions, Liana R. N. Schreiber, Marc N. Potenza, & Jon E. Grant - 17. Substance Abuse in Minority Populations, John Franklin - 18. Addiction in the Workplace, Laurence Westreich - 19. Forensic Approaches to Substances of Abuse, Avram H. Mack - 20. Patients with Chronic Pain and Opioid Misuse, Deborah L. Haller & Sidney H. Schnoll - 21. Substance Use among Older Adults, Steve Koh, Robert Gorney, Nicolas Badre, & Dilip Jeste 22. HIV/AIDS and Substance Use Disorders, Cheryl Ann Kennedy & Steven J. Schleifer - 23. Women and Substance Abuse, Dawn E. Sugarman, Christina Brezing, & Shelly F. Greenfield - 24. Substance Use Disorders in Adolescence, Oscar G. Bukstein & Yifrah Kaminer - V. Treatments for Addictions - 25. Matching and Differential Therapies: Providing Substance Abusers with Appropriate Treatment, Kathleen M. Carroll & Brian D. Kiluk - 26. Individual Psychodynamic Psychotherapy, Lance M. Dodes & Edward J. Khantzian - 27. Cognitive Therapy, Judith S. Beck, Bruce S. Liese, & Lisa M. Najavits - 28. Group Therapy, Self-Help Groups, and Network Therapy, Marc Galanter - 29. Family Therapy Approaches, Edward Kaufman - 30. Motivational Interviewing, Jennifer L. Smith, Kenneth M. Carpenter, R. Morgan Wain, & Edward V. Nunes - 31. Dialectical Behavior Therapy for Individuals with Borderline Personality Disorder and Substance Use Disorders, Dorian Hunter, M. Zachary Rosenthal, Thomas R. Lynch, and Marsha M. Linehan - 32. Psychopharmacological Treatments, Larissa J. Mooney & Elinore F. McCance-Katz - Index.

LC Subjects
Substance abuse.
Alcoholism.

Bibliography 103

Other Subjects	Psychology / Psychopathology / Addiction.
	Medical / Psychiatry / General.
	Social Science / Social Work.
	Psychology / Psychotherapy / Counseling.
	Medical / Nursing / Psychiatric.
Notes	Includes bibliographical references and index.

Club drugs and novel psychoactive substances: a clinical handbook

LCCN	2020026283
Type of material	Book
Personal name	Bowden-Jones, Owen, author.
Main title	Club drugs and novel psychoactive substances: a clinical handbook / Owen Bowden-Jones, Central North West London NHS Foundation Trust, Dima Abdulrahim, Central North West London NHS Foundation Trust.
Published/Produced	Cambridge, United Kingdom; New York, NY: Cambridge University Press, 2020.
Description	1 online resource
ISBN	9781911623106 (ebook)
	(paperback)
LC classification	RM316
Related names	Abdulrahim, Dima, author.
Summary	"Over the last decade the UK, Europe and beyond have seen a dramatic change in the patterns of illicit drug use, particularly in adolescents and those in their twenties for whom heroin and crack cocaine have steady lost popularity (Figure 1). While younger drug users continue to use established drugs such as powder cocaine and MDMA, some are attracted to a range of newly emerging drugs including so called club drugs and new psychoactive substances"-- Provided by publisher.
LC Subjects	Designer drugs.
	Psychotropic drugs.
	Drugs of abuse.
Notes	Includes bibliographical references and index.
Additional formats	Print version: Bowden-Jones, Owen. Club drugs and novel psychoactive substances Cambridge, United

Kingdom; New York, NY: Cambridge University Press, 2020. 9781911623090 (DLC) 2020026282

Club drugs and novel psychoactive substances: a clinical handbook
LCCN	2020026282
Type of material	Book
Personal name	Bowden-Jones, Owen, author.
Main title	Club drugs and novel psychoactive substances: a clinical handbook / Owen Bowden-Jones, Central North West London NHS Foundation Trust, Dima Abdulrahim, Central North West London NHS Foundation Trust.
Published/Produced	Cambridge, United Kingdom; New York, NY: Cambridge University Press, 2020.
ISBN	9781911623090 (paperback) (ebook)
LC classification	RM316 .B69 2020
Related names	Abdulrahim, Dima, author.
Summary	"Over the last decade the UK, Europe and beyond have seen a dramatic change in the patterns of illicit drug use, particularly in adolescents and those in their twenties for whom heroin and crack cocaine have steady lost popularity (Figure 1). While younger drug users continue to use established drugs such as powder cocaine and MDMA, some are attracted to a range of newly emerging drugs including so called club drugs and new psychoactive substances"-- Provided by publisher.
LC Subjects	Designer drugs. Psychotropic drugs. Drugs of abuse.
Notes	Includes bibliographical references and index.
Additional formats	Online version: Bowden-Jones, Owen. Club drugs and novel psychoactive substances Cambridge, United Kingdom; New York, NY: Cambridge University Press, 2020. 9781911623106 (DLC) 2020026283

Critical issues in alcohol and drugs of abuse testing
LCCN	2021304145
Type of material	Book
Main title	Critical issues in alcohol and drugs of abuse testing / edited by Amitava Dasgupta, PhD, Professor of Pathology and Laboratory Medicine, McGovern Medicine School, University of Texas Health Science Center at Houston, Houston, TX, United States.
Edition	Second edition.
Published/Produced	London, United Kingdom; San Diego: Academic Press, an imprint of Elsevier, [2019]
Description	xvii, 524 pages: illustrations; 28 cm
ISBN	9780128156070 paperback
	0128156074 paperback
LC classification	HV5823.5.U5 C75 2019
Portion of title	Alcohol and drugs of abuse testing
Related names	Dasgupta, Amitava, 1958- editor.
Summary	Critical Issues in Alcohol and Drugs of Abuse Testing, Second Edition, addresses the general principles and technological advances for measuring drugs and alcohol, along with the pitfalls of drugs of abuse testing. Many designer drugs, for example, are not routinely tested in drugs of abuse panels and may go undetected in a drug test. This updated edition is a must-have for clinical pathologists, toxicologists, clinicians, and medical review officers and regulators, bridging the gap between technical and clinical information. Topics of note include the monitoring of pain management drugs, bath salts, spices (synthetic marijuana), designer drugs and date rape drugs, and more.
Contents	Alcohol: pharmacokinetics, health benefits with moderate consumption and toxicity / Amitava Dasgupta - Alcohol analysis in various matrixes: clinical versus forensic testing / Steven C. Kazmierzak - Alcohol biomarkers: clinical issues and analytical methods / Joshua A. Bornhorst, Michael M. Mbughuni - Genetic markers related to alcohol use and abuse / Joshua A. Bornhorst, Gwendolyn

McMillin - Ethylene glycol and other glycols: analytical and interpretation issues / Uttam Garg, Jennifer Lowry, D. Adam Algren - Introduction to drugs of abuse / Loralie J. Langman, Christine L.H. Snozek - Legal aspects of drug testing in US military and civil courts / John F. Jemionek, Marilyn R. Past - Pharmacogenomics of drugs of abuse / Christine L.H. Snozek, Loralie J. Langman - Immunoassay design for screening of drugs of abuse / Pradip Datta - Issues of interferences with immunoassays used for screening of drugs of abuse in urine / Anu S. Maharjan, Kamisha L. Johnson-Davis - Point of care devices for drugs of abuse testing: limitations and pitfalls / Veronica Luzzi - Drugs of abuse screening and confirmation with lower cutoff values / Albert D. Fraser - Overview of analytical methods in drugs of abuse analysis: gas chromatography/mass spectrometry, liquid chromatography combined with tandem mass spectrometry and related methods / Alec Saitman - High-resolution mass spectometry: an emerging analytical method for drug testing / Michelle Wood - Confirmation methods for SAMHSA drugs and other commonly abused drugs / Justin Holler, Barry Levine - Critical issues when testing for amphetamine-type stimulants: pitfalls of immunoassay screening and mass spectrometric confirmation for amphetamines, methamphetamines, and designer amphetamines / Larry Broussard - Cocaine, crack cocaine and ethanol: a deadly mix / Eric T. Shimomura, George F. Jackson, Buddha Dev Paul - Drug assisted sexual assaults: toxicology, fatality and analytical challenge / Matthew D. Krasowski - Overview of common designer drugs / Lilian H.J. Richter, Markus R. Meyer, Hans H. Maurer - New psychoactive substances: an overview / Laura Mercolini - Review of bath salts on illicit drug market / Michele Protti - Review of synthetic cannabinoids on illicit drug market / Mahmoud A. ElSohly, Sohail Ahmed, Shahbaz W. Gul, Waseem

	Gul - Application of liquid chromatography combined with high resolution mass spectrometry for urine drug testing / Olef Bek, Alexia Rylski, Niclas Nikolai Stephanson - Forensic toxicology in death investigation / Hannah Kastenbaum, Lori Proe, Lauren Dvorscak - Drug testing in pain management / Gary M. Reisfield, Roger L. Bertholf - How do people try to beat drugs test? Effects of synthetic urine, substituted urine, diluted urine and in vitro urinary adulterants on drugs of abuse testing / Shanlin Fu - When hospital toxicology report is negative in a suspected overdosed patient: strategy of comprehensive drug screen using liquid chromatography combined with mass spectrometry / Ernest D. Lykissa - Testing of drugs in oral fluid, sweat, hair and nail: analytical, interpretative and specimen adulteration issues / Uttam Garg, Carl Cooley - Advances in meconium analysis for assessment of neonatal drug exposure / Steven W. Cotten - Analytical true positive drug tests due to use of prescription and non-prescription medications / Matthew D. Krasowski, Tai C. Kwong - Analytical true positive: poppy seed products and opiate analysis / Amitava Dasgupta - Miscellaneous issues: paper money contaminated with cocaine and other drugs, cocaine containing herbal teas, passive exposure of marijuana, ingestion of hemp oil and occupational exposure to controlled substances / Amitava Dasgupta - Abuse of magic mushroom, peyote cactus, LSD, khat, and volatiles / Amitava Dasgupta - Performance enhancing drugs in sports / Brian D. Ahrens, Anthony W. Butch.
LC Subjects	Alcohol--Toxicology. Alcohol in the body--Testing. Drug testing--United States.
Other Subjects	Substance Abuse Detection--methods Chemistry Techniques, Analytical--methods Alcohol--Toxicology. Alcohol in the body--Testing.

Notes	Drug testing. United States. Includes bibliographical references and index.
Additional formats	ebook version: 9780128156087

Dopeworld: adventures in the global drug trade

LCCN	2020010724
Type of material	Book
Personal name	Vorobyov, Niko, author.
Main title	Dopeworld: adventures in the global drug trade / Niko Vorobyov.
Edition	First U.S. edition.
Published/Produced	New York: St. Martin's Press, 2020. ©2019
ISBN	9781250270016 (hardcover) (ebook)
LC classification	HV5801.V65 2020
Summary	"Just as Anthony Bourdain did for the world of food, in Dopeworld, writer Niko Vorobyov travels the globe to find out more about the war on drugs and how it affects global politics and our day-to-day lives. Dopeworld is a bold and intoxicating journey into the world of drugs. From the cocaine farms in South America to the streets of Manila, this book traces the emergence of psychoactive substances and our intimate relationship with them. With unparalleled access to drug lords, cartel leaders, street dealers and government officials, Vorobyov attempts to shine a light on the dark underbelly of the drug world. At once a bold piece of reportage and a hugely entertaining and perverse travelogue, with echoes of Gomorrah and Fear and Loathing in Las Vegas, Dopeworld reveals how drug use is at the heart of our history, our lives, and our world"-- Provided by publisher.
LC Subjects	Drug traffic. Drug dealers. Drug abuse. Drug control.

Bibliography

Notes	Includes bibliographical references.

Drug use and harm reduction

LCCN	2020447089
Type of material	Book
Main title	Drug use and harm reduction / edited by Justin Healey.
Published/Produced	Thirroul, NSW, Australia: The Spinney Press, [2020] ©2020
Description	60 pages: color illustrations; 30 cm.
ISBN	9781922274069 (paperback) (PDF)
LC classification	HV5840.A8 D784 2020
Related names	Healey, Justin, editor.
Summary	Harm reduction entails policies, programs and practices aimed at reducing the harms associated with the use of psychoactive drugs in people who are unwilling or unable to stop. The focus is on the prevention of harm, rather than on the prevention of drug use itself. Harm reduction has been a principle of Australia's approach to drug use for several decades. However, recent overdose deaths and hospitalisations at music festivals have highlighted the clear harms of illicit drug use and prompted a debate over the introduction of pill testing, with political leaders being reluctant to implement the measure. This book explores the ethical, legal and medical pros and cons in the debate, with a topical focus on pill testing. Does pill testing give young people a false sense of security and promote further risky drug use, when there is really no safe level at which these substances can be taken? Or are harm reduction approaches such as pill testing and needle and syringe programs simply about saving lives and giving people a safety net? In a perfect world, no one would risk their lives by taking party drugs but in reality, is harm reduction too bitter a pill to swallow?-- Source other than Library of Congress.
LC Subjects	Drug control--Australia.

	Harm reduction--Australia.
	Psychotropic drugs--Australia.
	Drug traffic--Australia.
	Drug abuse--Australia.
Notes	Includes bibliographical references and index.
Series	Issues in society; volume 453

Drugs in American society

LCCN	2014008162
Type of material	Book
Personal name	Goode, Erich.
Main title	Drugs in American society / Erich Goode, Stony Brook University.
Edition	Ninth Edition.
Published/Produced	Dubuque: McGraw-Hill Education, 2014.
Description	xvi, 472 pages: illustration: 24 cm.
Links	Table of contents only http://www.loc.gov/catdir/enhancements/fy1408/2014008162-t.html
	Publisher description http://www.loc.gov/catdir/enhancements/fy1408/2014008162-d.html
	Contributor biographical information http://www.loc.gov/catdir/enhancements/fy1408/2014008162-b.html
ISBN	9780078026591 (paperback: alk. paper)
LC classification	HV5825.G63 2014
Summary	"Drugs in American Society is a sociological introduction to the use of psychoactive substances in the United States that takes the focus out of the lab and onto the street. Throughout the book, personal accounts tell the stories of drug use and the impact that it has on the lives of users. The book also contrasts the image of drugs in society, particularly in the news media, and the reality of drug use itself"--Provided by publisher.
	"A study of drug use is also crucial from a policy standpoint. It is in fact, a life-or-death proposition. Drug abuse can kill. In addition, drug use, whether directly or indirectly, often spawns a swarming host of sub-lethal problems: disease, poor quality of life,

	enslavement to a chemical, lower academic and job performance, victimization by robbers, rapists, and all other manner of violent offenders, the fear by residents of a community for their safety, the fear of leaving their homes at night, and subversion of friendship, romantic, and family relations. In the United States alone, smoking claims over 400,000 victims a year--and gradually, in response to studies on the medical harms of smoking, year by year, smokers are giving up the deadly habit"-- Provided by publisher.
Contents	Preface and Acknowledgments *Part One: A History of Drug Use and Drug Control* 1) A History of Drug Use 2) A History of Drug Control *Part Two: Three Perspectives on Drug Use* 3) The Pharmacological Perspective 4) The Sociologist Looks at Drug Use 5) Drugs in the Media *Part Three: Methods, Data, Theories* 6) Studying Drug Use 7) Explaining Drug Use *Part Four: Drugs and Their Use* 8) Legal Drugs Use: Alcohol and Tobacco 9) Prescription Drugs 10) Marijuana, LSD, and Club Drugs 11) Stimulants: Amphetamine, Methamphetamine, Cocaine and Crack 12) Heroin and the *Narcotics Part Five: Drugs, Crime, and Drug Control* 13) Drugs and Crime 14) Trafficking in Illicit Drugs 15) Law Enforcement, Drug Courts, and Drug Treatment 16) Legalization, Decriminalization, and Harm Reduction Glossary References Photo Credits Name Index Subject Index.
LC Subjects	Drug abuse--United States.
	Drugs--United States.
	Drug utilization--United States.
	Drug abuse and crime--United States.
Other Subjects	Social Science / Sociology / General.
Notes	Includes bibliographical references and index.

Drugs, behavior, and modern society

LCCN	2021058634
Type of material	Book
Personal name	Levinthal, Charles F., 1945-, author.

Bibliography

Main title	Drugs, behavior, and modern society / Charles F. Levinthal, Professor Emeritus, Hofstra University.
Edition	Ninth edition.
Published/Produced	Hoboken, NJ: Pearson Education, Inc., [2023]
ISBN	9780135385340 (paperback)
	9780135385883 (spiral bound)
	(epub)
LC classification	HV5801.L49 2023
Summary	"I welcome all of you to the Ninth Edition of Drugs, Behavior, and Modern Society. As always, the overarching goal has been to provide a valuable learning experience and a greater understanding of the complex world of drug-taking behavior. Throughout the chapters of this book, the focus will be on the relevance of drugs and drug-taking behavior on your daily lives as well as the contemporary society in which we live. There is no need for a background in biology, sociology, Psychology, or chemistry to receive benefit from the contents of this book. The only requirement is a sense of curiosity about the range of drugs that affect our minds and our bodies and a concern about the social and personal challenges that drugs bring to our daily lives. These challenges can be framed in terms of three fundamental themes of understanding: Understanding the patterns of drug-taking behavior throughout history Present-day issues concerning drug misuse and abuse are issues that society has confronted for a long time. Drugs and drug-taking behavior are consequences of a particularly human need to feel stronger, more alert, calmer, more distant and dissociated from our surroundings, or simply to feel good. It is the misuse and abuse of chemical substances to achieve these ends that have resulted in major problems in the United States and around the world. Understanding the diversity of psychoactive drugs in our society There is an enormous diversity among drugs that affect the mind and the body. There is a great need to educate ourselves not only about

drugs such as cocaine, amphetamines, heroin, hallucinogens, and marijuana but also about drugs that are legally sanctioned and readily available to us, specifically alcohol and nicotine. Drugs, Behavior, and Modern Society is a comprehensive survey of all types of psychoactive drugs, addressing the issues of drug-taking behavior from psychological, biological, and sociological perspectives. Understanding the impact of society on drug-related issues in our lives - Like it or not, the decision to use drugs is one of life's choices within our contemporary society, regardless of your racial, ethnic, or religious background, how much money you have, where you live, how much education you have acquired, your age or gender identity. As has been demonstrated through our collective experiences during the days of the COVID pandemic, our behaviors will be continually influenced by changes in the social environment around us. As far as the contents of this new edition are concerned, let's say that there are some things that are old and somethings that are new. On the one hand, the Ninth Edition of Drugs, Behavior, and Modern Society continues to maintain standards of clarity, readability, comprehensiveness, and organization that have been set by previous editions, as well as a commitment to the importance of historical storytelling as a meaningful context to the technical material in the chapters. On the other hand, the story of drug-taking behavior through the years is like a breathless ride on a high-speed train with twists and turns and unknown territory just around the bend. It is obvious that certain patterns of drug-taking behavior and associated social issues have changed dramatically since the previous edition of this book. In fact, there are a number of subjects ad-dressed in the new edition that hardly existed at the time the Eighth Edition was released. Some examples include: the widespread prevalence of nicotine vaping and the use of e-cigarettes in general (Chapter 10), advancements in medical applications of cannabis (Chapter 7), and the impactful nature of the opioid abuse epidemic made worse by the availability of synthetic opioids such as fentanyl (Chapter 4). In addition, there have been groundbreaking developments in understanding the neurochemical basis for behavioral addiction (Chapter 3). [Insert Screen break] Content Highlights As you will see, chapters about particular drugs have been grouped not in terms of their pharmacological or chemical characteristics but, rather, in terms of how readily accessible they are to the general public and today's societal attitudes toward their use. The last section of the book concerns itself with prevention and treatment. In addition, several special features throughout the book will enhance your experience as a reader and serve as learning aids. This text is available in a variety of formats-digital and print. To learn more about our programs, pricing options, and customization, visit www.pearsonhighered.com. Beyond the subject matter, however, there are several features contained in the book itself that are new to this edition"-- Provided by publisher.

LC Subjects	Drugs.
	Drug abuse.
	Drugs--Physiological effect.
	Psychotropic drugs.
	Psychopharmacology.
Notes	Includes bibliographical references and index.
Additional formats	Online version: Levinthal, Charles F., 1945- Drugs, behavior, and modern society. Ninth edition Hoboken, NJ: Pearson Education, Inc., [2023] 9780135385913 (DLC) 2021058635

Drugs, behavior, and modern society

LCCN	2021058635
Type of material	Book
Personal name	Levinthal, Charles F., 1945-, author.

Main title	Drugs, behavior, and modern society / Charles F. Levinthal, Professor Emeritus, Hofstra University.
Edition	Ninth edition.
Published/Produced	Hoboken, NJ: Pearson Education, Inc., [2023]
Description	1 online resource
ISBN	9780135385913 (epub)
	(paperback)
	(spiral bound)
LC classification	HV5801
Summary	"I welcome all of you to the Ninth Edition of Drugs, Behavior, and Modern Society. As always, the overarching goal has been to provide a valuable learning experience and a greater understanding of the complex world of drug-taking behavior. Throughout the chapters of this book, the focus will be on the relevance of drugs and drug-taking behavior on your daily lives as well as the contemporary society in which we live. There is no need for a background in biology, sociology, Psychology, or chemistry to receive benefit from the contents of this book. The only requirement is a sense of curiosity about the range of drugs that affect our minds and our bodies and a concern about the social and personal challenges that drugs bring to our daily lives. These challenges can be framed in terms of three fundamental themes of understanding: Understanding the patterns of drug-taking behavior throughout history Present-day issues concerning drug misuse and abuse are issues that society has confronted for a long time. Drugs and drug-taking behavior are consequences of a particularly human need to feel stronger, more alert, calmer, more distant and dissociated from our surroundings, or simply to feel good. It is the misuse and abuse of chemical substances to achieve these ends that have resulted in major problems in the United States and around the world. Understanding the diversity of psychoactive drugs in our society There is an enormous diversity among drugs that affect the mind and the body. There

is a great need to educate ourselves not only about drugs such as cocaine, amphetamines, heroin, hallucinogens, and marijuana but also about drugs that are legally sanctioned and readily available to us, specifically alcohol and nicotine. Drugs, Behavior, and Modern Society is a comprehensive survey of all types of psychoactive drugs, addressing the issues of drug-taking behavior from psychological, biological, and sociological perspectives. Understanding the impact of society on drug-related issues in our lives - Like it or not, the decision to use drugs is one of life's choices within our contemporary society, regardless of your racial, ethnic, or religious background, how much money you have, where you live, how much education you have acquired, your age or gender identity. As has been demonstrated through our collective experiences during the days of the COVID pandemic, our behaviors will be continually influenced by changes in the social environment around us. As far as the contents of this new edition are concerned, let's say that there are some things that are old and somethings that are new. On the one hand, the Ninth Edition of Drugs, Behavior, and Modern Society continues to maintain standards of clarity, readability, comprehensiveness, and organization that have been set by previous editions, as well as a commitment to the importance of historical storytelling as a meaningful context to the technical material in the chapters. On the other hand, the story of drug-taking behavior through the years is like a breathless ride on a high-speed train with twists and turns and unknown territory just around the bend. It is obvious that certain patterns of drug-taking behavior and associated social issues have changed dramatically since the previous edition of this book. In fact, there are a number of subjects ad-dressed in the new edition that hardly existed at the time the Eighth Edition was released. Some examples include: the widespread prevalence of nicotine vaping and the

	use of e-cigarettes in general (Chapter 10), advancements in medical applications of cannabis (Chapter 7), and the impactful nature of the opioid abuse epidemic made worse by the availability of synthetic opioids such as fentanyl (Chapter 4). In addition, there have been groundbreaking developments in understanding the neurochemical basis for behavioral addiction (Chapter 3). [Insert Screen break] Content Highlights As you will see, chapters about particular drugs have been grouped not in terms of their pharmacological or chemical characteristics but, rather, in terms of how readily accessible they are to the general public and today's societal attitudes toward their use. The last section of the book concerns itself with prevention and treatment. In addition, several special features throughout the book will enhance your experience as a reader and serve as learning aids. This text is available in a variety of formats-digital and print. To learn more about our programs, pricing options, and customization, visit www.pearsonhighered.com. Beyond the subject matter, however, there are several features contained in the book itself that are new to this edition"-- Provided by publisher.
LC Subjects	Drugs.
	Drug abuse.
	Drugs--Physiological effect.
	Psychotropic drugs.
	Psychopharmacology.
Notes	Includes bibliographical references and index.
Additional formats	Print version: Levinthal, Charles F., 1945-. Drugs, behavior, and modern society Ninth edition. Hoboken, NJ: Pearson Education, Inc., [2023] 9780135385340 (DLC) 2021058634

Dual markets: comparative approaches to regulation
LCCN	2019758096
Type of material	Book

Main title	Dual Markets: Comparative Approaches to Regulation / edited by Ernesto U. Savona, Mark A.R. Kleiman, Francesco Calderoni.
Edition	1st ed. 2017.
Published/Produced	Cham: Springer International Publishing: Imprint: Springer, 2017.
Description	1 online resource (XVIII, 402 pages 12 illustrations, 10 illustrations in color.) PDF
ISBN	9783319653617
Related names	Calderoni, Francesco. editor. Kleiman, Mark, 1951-2019, editor. Savona, Ernesto U. editor.
Summary	This comprehensive volume analyzes dual markets for regulated substances and services, and aims to provide a framework for their effective regulation. A "dual market" refers to the existence of both a legal and an illegal market for a regulated product or service (for example, prescription drugs). These regulations exist in various countries for a mix of public health, historical, political and cultural reasons. Allowing the legal market to thrive, while trying to eliminate the illegal market, provides a unique challenge for governments and law enforcement. Broken down into nine main sections, the book studies comparative international policies for regulating these "dual markets" from a historical, legal, and cultural perspective. It includes an analysis of the markets for psychoactive substances that are illegal in most countries (such as marijuana, cocaine, opiods and amphetimines), psychoactive substances which are legal in most countries and where consumption is widespread (such as alcohol and tobacco), and services that are generally regulated or illegal (such as sports betting, the sex trade, and gambling). For each of these nine types of markets, contributions focus on the relationship between regulation, the emerging illegal market, and the resulting overall access to these services. This work

	aims to provide a comprehensive framework from a historical, cultural, and comparative international perspective. It will be of interest to researchers in criminology and criminal justice, particularly with an interest in organized crime, as well as related fields such as sociology, public policy, international relations, and public health.
LC Subjects	Conflict of laws. Criminology. Health promotion. Private international law.
Other Subjects	Criminology and Criminal Justice, general. Health Promotion and Disease Prevention. Private International Law, International & Foreign Law, Comparative Law.
Additional formats	Print version: Dual markets: comparative approaches for regulation 9783319653600 (DLC) 2017955079 Printed edition: 9783319653600 Printed edition: 9783319653624 Printed edition: 9783319880068

Essential substances: a cultural history of intoxicants

LCCN	2022304707
Type of material	Book
Personal name	Rudgley, Richard, 1961- author.
Main title	Essential substances: a cultural history of intoxicants / Richard Rudgley.
Published/Produced	[London?]: Arktos Media Ltd., 2014.
Description	xviii, 182 pages: illustrations; 23 cm
ISBN	9781910524091 1910524093 9781910524084 1910524085
LC classification	GN411 .R83 2014
Variant title	Subtitle on jacket: Intoxicants in society
Summary	"Richard Rudgely's first book, Essential Substances, was the winner of the British Museum Prometheus Award and hailed as a masterpiece by the Director of Harvard Botanical Museum, the world's leading

Contents	authority on hallucinogenic plants. It is still one of the few books to have explored the role of drugs in the religious, political, economic and sexual life of our species from prehistory to the present day ... Added for this edition is a new appendix, 'A Psychoactive Bestiary'."--Jacket.

Contents: Foreword / by William Emboden - Introduction - Stone age alchemy - Frozen tombs and fly-agaric men - The mystery of Haoma - American dreams - The alchemists of Afek - Lucifer's garden - Stimulating society - Conclusion - Appendix. Psychoactive bestiary.

LC Subjects: Psychotropic drugs--Cross-cultural studies.
Narcotics--Cross-cultural studies.
Drinking of alcoholic beverages--Cross-cultural studies.
Psychotropic drugs--History.
Narcotics--History.
Drinking of alcoholic beverages--History.

Other Subjects: Drinking of alcoholic beverages.
Narcotics.
Psychotropic drugs.

Form/Genre: Cross-cultural studies.
History.

Notes: Also published under title: The alchemy of culture: intoxicants in society.
Includes bibliographical references (pages 171-181).

Essentials of pharmacology for anesthesia, pain medicine, and critical care

LCCN: 2014948072
Type of material: Book
Main title: Essentials of pharmacology for anesthesia, pain medicine, and critical care / Alan David Kaye, Adam M. Kaye, Richard D. Urman, editors.
Published/Produced: New York: Springer, [2015]
©2015
Description: xxii, 904 pages: illustrations (some color); 24 cm
ISBN: 9781461489474 (print: alk. paper)

LC classification	1461489474 (print: alk. paper) RD81.E775 2015
Related names	Kaye, Alan David. editor. Kaye, Adam M., editor. Urman, Richard D., editor.
Summary	In anesthesiology, pain medicine, and critical care, practitioners at all levels need help to stay current with the continually evolving drug knowledge-base, and trainees need tools to prepare for in-training and board exams that increasingly test their knowledge of pharmacology. This practical book is aimed at both readerships. It features a unique and practical chapter on the United States Food and Drug Administration (FDA) "black box" warnings that describe what safety precautions should be taken with commonly used drugs. The editors and contributors are pharmacology experts representing a cross-section of clinical specialties and institutions in the United States and include pharmacologists, pharmacists, as well as physicians. - Source other than Library of Congress.
Contents	Part I. Basic Pharmacologic Principles - 1. Pharmacokinetics and Pharmacodynamics of Anesthetics - 2. A Review of Mechanisms of Inhalational Anesthetic Agents - 3. Pharmacokinetics, pharmacodynamics and physical properties of Inhalational agents - 4. Principles of Total Intravenous Anesthesia - 5. Perioperative Considerations in Pharmacology - Part II. Drug Classes - 6. Anesthetic Induction Agents - 7. Analgesics: Opiate agonists, mixed agonist/ antagonists and antagonists for acute pain management - 8. Analgesics: Opioids for chronic pain management and surgical considerations - 9. Nonopioid Analgesic and Adjunct Drugs - 10. Benzodiazepines and muscle relaxants - 11. Pharmacology of Local Anesthetics - 12. Neuromuscular Blockers - 13. Reversal agents - 14. Drugs acting on the autonomic nervous system - 15. Antihypertensives, diuretics and antidysrhythmics - 16. Peripheral

vasodilators - 17. Nitric oxide and Pulmonary Vasodilators - 18. Asthma and COPD agents - 19. Hormones, Part 1: Thyroid and Corticosteroid Hormones - 20. Hormones, Part 2: Insulin and Other glucose controlling Medications - 21. Antacids, Gastrointestinal Prokinetics, And Proton Pump Inhibitors - 22. Histamine modulators - 23. Central Nervous System Stimulants - 24. Anticoagulant drugs - 25. Hemostatic Agents - 26. Blood, Blood Products, and Substitutes - 27. Antipyretics: Acetaminophen, Arachidonic Acid Agents, Cox1 and Cox2 Inhibitors - 28. Antiemetic Agents - 29. Antiepileptics agents - 30. Neuropharmacologic agents for neurologic conditions - 31. Chemotherapeutic Agents - 32. Antimicrobial Agents - 33. Herbals medications and vitamin supplements - 34. Minerals and electrolytes - 35. Disinfection agents and antiseptics - 36. Psychopharmacologic agents and psychiatric drug considerations - 37. Cocaine, Methamphetamine, MDMA and Heroin - Part III. Clinical Subspecialties - 38. Cardiac surgery - 39. The Intensive Care Unit - 40. Enteral and parenteral nutrition - 41. Obstetrics - 42. Pediatrics - 43. Neurologic Surgery - 44. Liver disease and liver transplantation - Part IV. Special Topics - 45. Black Box FDA warnings and legal implications - 46. Drug-Induced QT Prolongation - 47. Drugs and Cancer Propagation - 48. Lipid Lowering Agents - 49. Serotonin Syndrome - Part V. New Vistas in Pharmacology - 50. Novel Psychoactive Substances: synthetic cathinones and cannabinoid receptor agonists - 51. New Vistas in Anesthetics, IV Induction Agents - 52. New Vistas In Neuromuscular Blockers - 53. Patient-Controlled Analgesia: The Importance of Effector Site Pharmacokinetics - 54. Understanding anesthesia-induced memory loss - 55. Novel Targets of Current Analgesic Drug Development.

LC Subjects Pharmacology.

Other Subjects	Anesthesiology. Anesthesia adjuvants. Critical care medicine. Pain medicine. Anesthetics--pharmacology. Analgesics--pharmacology. Critical Care. Pain--drug therapy. Pharmacology. Medicine & Public Health. Intensive / Critical Care Medicine. Anesthesiology. Critical care medicine. Medicine. Pain medicine.
Notes	Includes bibliographical references and index.

Fentanyl, Inc.: how rogue chemists are creating the deadliest wave of the opioid epidemic

LCCN	2019033267
Type of material	Book
Personal name	Westhoff, Ben, author.
Main title	Fentanyl, Inc.: how rogue chemists are creating the deadliest wave of the opioid epidemic / Ben Westhoff.
Edition	First edition. First Grove Atlantic hardcover edition.
Published/Produced	New York: Atlantic Monthly Press, 2019. ©2019
Description	341 pages; 24 cm
ISBN	9780802127433 (hardcover) (ebook)
LC classification	RC568.O45 W47 2019
Summary	"A deeply human story, Fentanyl, Inc. is the first deep-dive investigation of a hazardous and illicit industry that has created a worldwide epidemic, ravaging communities and overwhelming and confounding government agencies that are challenged to combat it. 'A whole new crop of

	chemicals is radically changing the recreational drug landscape,' writes Ben Westhoff. 'These are known as Novel Psychoactive Substances (NPS) and they include replacements for known drugs like heroin, cocaine, ecstasy, and marijuana. They are synthetic, made in a laboratory, and are much more potent than traditional drugs'-and all-too-often tragically lethal. Drugs like fentanyl, K2, and Spice were all originally conceived in legitimate laboratories. Their formulas were then hijacked and manufactured by rogue chemists, largely in China, who change their molecular structures to stay ahead of the law, making the drugs' effects impossible to predict. Westhoff has infiltrated this world, tracking down the little-known scientists who invented these drugs and inadvertently killed thousands. He visits the factories in China from which these drugs emanate, providing startling and original reporting on how China's vast chemical industry operates, and how the Chinese government subsidizes it. He poignantly chronicles the lives of addicted users and dealers, families of victims, law enforcement officers, and underground drug awareness organizers in the U.S. and Europe. Together they represent the shocking and riveting full anatomy of a calamity we are just beginning to understand and the new strategies slowly emerging that may provide essential long-term solutions to the drug crisis that has affected so many"-- Provided by publisher.
LC Subjects	Designer drugs. Fentanyl. Opioid abuse--United States. Drug addiction--United States. Drug abuse--Fentanyl. Addictions--Fentanyl. Designer drugs--Fentanyl. Drug traffic--China.
Notes	Includes bibliographical references (pages 291-328) and index.

Bibliography

Forensic toxicology: drug use and misuse

LCCN	2016462073
Type of material	Book
Main title	Forensic toxicology: drug use and misuse / edited by Susannah Davies, LTG, London, UK, Atholl Johnston, Queen Mary University of London, UK, David Holt, St George's, University of London, UK.
Published/Produced	Cambridge: Royal Society of Chemistry, [2016] ©2016
Description	xx, 569 pages: illustrations (some color); 24 cm.
ISBN	1782621563 9781782621560
LC classification	HV8073.F6133 2016
Related names	Davies, Susannah, editor. Johnston, Atholl, editor. Holt, David W., editor.
Summary	The text begins with an in-depth discussion of pharmaco-epidemiology, including information on the value of nationwide databases in forensic toxicology. The use and abuse of drugs in driving, sport and the workplace are then discussed by industry experts who are conducting case work in their fields. Not only are new drug groups discussed (NPS), but also their constantly changing impact on drug legislation. Synthetic cannabinoids, khat and mephodrone are discussed in detail. Following a section devoted to legislation and defence, readers will find comprehensive chapters covering sample choice reflecting the increasing use of hair and oral fluid, also the less commonly used sweat and nail analysis. New and old case examples are compared and contrasted in the final part of the book, which will enable readers to understand how drugs impact on each other and how the interpretative outcome of a case are dependent on many aspects. - Provided by publisher.
Contents	Introduction to forensic toxicology and the value of a nationwide database / Alan Wayne Jones - Forensic pharmacology / Nigel J. Langford - The role of

amnesty bins in understanding the pattern of recreational drugs and novel psychoactive substances being used within a locality / David M. Wood and Paul I. Dargan - Contamination of water with drugs and metabolites / Victoria Hilborne - Understanding the utility of analysis of anonymous pooled urine from standalone urinals in detecting and monitoring recreational drug use / David M. Wood and Paul I. Dargan - Mephedrone and new psychoactive substances / Simon Elliott - Novel psychoactives in New Zealand / Samantha J. Coward and Hilary J. Hamnett - Cannabis and synthetic cannabinoids / Kim Wolff - Khat - chewing it over: continuing "cultural cement," cardiac challenge ot catalyst for change? / John Martin Corkery - Role of analytical screening in the management and assessment of acute recreational drug toxicity / David M. Wood and Paul I. Dargan - Workplace drug testing / Simon Walker - Current issues in human sport drug testing: clenbuterol, erythropoietin and xenon / A.Y. Kicman, D.A. Cowan and I. Gavrilović - Drugs and driving / Kim Wolff - Alcohol technical defences in road traffic casework / Mike Scott-Ham - New psychoactive substances and the criminal law / Rudi Fortson - Scheduling of drugs in the United States / Jeffery Hackett - Drug legislation in New Zealand / Keith Bedford - Use of reference materials in toxicology / Jennifer Button - Nail analysis in forensic toxicology / Nikolas P. Lemos - Hair testing in forensic toxicology / Donna M. Cave and Robert Kingston - Drugs in oral fluid / Peter Akrill - Sweat as an alternative biological matrix / Nadia De Giovanni - Smart drugs / Angela Wing Gar Kwan - Substandard and counterfeit medicines / Badr Aljohani - Detection of drugs and drug metabolites from fingerprints / Paula García Calavia and David A. Russell - Investigating drug metabolism of new psychoactive substances using human liver preparations and animal studies / Markus R. Meyer

	and Hans H. Maurer - Case examples and discussion / John Slaughter.
LC Subjects	Chemistry, Forensic.
	Forensic toxicology.
	Drug testing.
Other Subjects	Forensic Toxicology--methods.
	Substance Abuse Detection.
	Drug Misuse.
	Toxicological Phenomena.
	Chemistry, Forensic.
	Drug testing.
	Forensic toxicology.
Notes	Includes bibliographical references and index.

Gas chromatography: history, methods and applications

LCCN	2020000182
Type of material	Book
Main title	Gas chromatography: history, methods and applications / [edited by Percy Henrichon].
Published/Produced	New York: Nova Science Publishers, Inc., [2019]
Description	1 online resource
ISBN	9781536173529 (adobe pdf)
	(paperback)
LC classification	TP156.C5
Related names	Henrichon, Percy, editor.
Summary	"Gas Chromatography: History, Methods and Applications focuses on the main applications of gas chromatography in clinical and forensic toxicology, mainly in the determination of drugs of abuse including the new psychoactive substances in several types of biological matrices. The authors go on to investigated the analysis of gaseous or volatile substances using sensor gas chromatography equipped with a semiconductor gas sensor detector. The simplicity, ease of handling, and high sensitivity of this method allow results to be obtained rapidly, which may provide valuable information for forensic diagnosis. This compilation addresses the way in which food adulteration practices are potentially

Contents	harmful to human health and so food safety and authenticity constitute an important issue in food chemistry. The chemical composition of foodstuffs is an excellent indicator of quality, origin, authenticity and/or adulteration. The concluding study aims to determine the organic compounds of vinasse through gas chromatography-mass spectrometry GC-MS. Vinasse is a byproduct of ethanol and poses long-term risk to public health because of its persistent and toxic nature"-- Provided by publisher. The role of gas chromatography in clinical and forensic toxicology / Ana Y. Simão, Mónica Antunes, Joana Gonçalves, Sofia Soares, Teresa Castro, Tiago Rosado, Débora Caramelo, Mário Barroso, André R.T.S. Araújo, Jesus Rodilla, and Eugenia Gallardo - Application of sensor gas chromatography in forensic medicine / Hiroshi Kinoshita, Naoko Tanaka, Mostofa Jamal, Asuka Ito, Mitsuru Kumihashi, Tadayoshi Yamashita, Shoji Kimura, Yasuhiko Kimura, Kunihiko Tsutsui, Shuji Matsubara and Kiyoshi Ameno - Trends of gas chromatography-mass spectrometry techniques in food authentication / Oscar Núñez - Gas chromatography-mass spectrometry analysis of sugarcane vinasse / Mohamed A. Fagier and Mona O. Abdalrhman.
LC Subjects	Gas chromatography--Industrial applications.
Notes	Includes bibliographical references and index.
Additional formats	Print version: Gas chromatography New York: Nova Science Publishers, Inc., [2019] 9781536173505 (DLC) 2020000181
Series	Analytical chemistry and microchemistry

Gas chromatography: history, methods and applications

LCCN	2020000181
Type of material	Book
Main title	Gas chromatography: history, methods and applications / [edited by Percy Henrichon].
Published/Produced	New York: Nova Science Publishers, Inc., [2019]
Description	x, 201 pages: ill.; 22 cm.

ISBN	9781536173505 (paperback)
	(adobe pdf)
LC classification	TP156.C5.G29 2019
Related names	Henrichon, Percy, editor.
Summary	"Gas Chromatography: History, Methods and Applications focuses on the main applications of gas chromatography in clinical and forensic toxicology, mainly in the determination of drugs of abuse including the new psychoactive substances in several types of biological matrices. The authors go on to investigated the analysis of gaseous or volatile substances using sensor gas chromatography equipped with a semiconductor gas sensor detector. The simplicity, ease of handling, and high sensitivity of this method allow results to be obtained rapidly, which may provide valuable information for forensic diagnosis. This compilation addresses the way in which food adulteration practices are potentially harmful to human health and so food safety and authenticity constitute an important issue in food chemistry. The chemical composition of foodstuffs is an excellent indicator of quality, origin, authenticity and/or adulteration. The concluding study aims to determine the organic compounds of vinasse through gas chromatography-mass spectrometry GC-MS. Vinasse is a byproduct of ethanol and poses long-term risk to public health because of its persistent and toxic nature"-- Provided by publisher.
Contents	The role of gas chromatography in clinical and forensic toxicology / Ana Y. Simão, Mónica Antunes, Joana Gonçalves, Sofia Soares, Teresa Castro, Tiago Rosado, Débora Caramelo, Mário Barroso, André R.T.S. Araújo, Jesus Rodilla, and Eugenia Gallardo -- Application of sensor gas chromatography in forensic medicine / Hiroshi Kinoshita, Naoko Tanaka, Mostofa Jamal, Asuka Ito, Mitsuru Kumihashi, Tadayoshi Yamashita, Shoji Kimura, Yasuhiko Kimura, Kunihiko Tsutsui, Shuji Matsubara and Kiyoshi Ameno -- Trends of gas chromatography-

	mass spectrometry techniques in food authentication / Oscar Núñez - Gas chromatography-mass spectrometry analysis of sugarcane vinasse / Mohamed A.Fagier and Mona O. Abdalrhman.
LC Subjects	Gas chromatography--Industrial applications.
Notes	Includes bibliographical references and index.
Additional formats	Online version: Gas chromatography New York: Nova Science Publishers, Inc., [2019] 9781536173529 (DLC) 2020000182
Series	Analytical chemistry and microchemistry

Handbook of novel psychoactive substances: what clinicians should know about NPS

LCCN	2018027784
Type of material	Book
Main title	Handbook of novel psychoactive substances: what clinicians should know about NPS / edited by Ornella Corazza and Andres Roman-Urrestarazu.
Published/Produced	New York, NY: Routledge, 2019.
Description	1 online resource.
ISBN	9781351655521 (epub) 9781315158082 (E-book) 9781351655538 (pdf)
LC classification	RM315
Related names	Corazza, Ornella, editor. Roman-Urrestarazu, Andres, editor.
Contents	Overcoming the NPS challenge: an introduction / Ornella Corazza & Andres Roman-Urrestarazu - The need for clinical guidelines on NPS: NEPTUNE / Owen Bowden-Jones & Dima Abdulrahim - NPS: epidemiology, user group characteristics, patterns, motives and problems / Máté Kapitány-Fövény, Ariel M. Weinstein & Zsolt Demetrovics - The NPS crisis in British prisons / Shanna Marrinan, Giuseppe Bersani & Ornella Corazza - Current trends in performance and image enhancing substance use among gym goers, exercisers and athletes / Neha P. Ainsworth, Jake Shelley & Andrea Petróczi - NPS in emergency rooms: dealing with aggressiveness and

psychomotor agitation / Carla Morganti, Attilio Negri, Laura Cazzaniga, Riccardo C. Gatti & Franca Davanzo - A sentinel and design model of evidence collection on acute drug and NPS toxicity: the euroden plus project / Luke de la Rue, David M. Wood & Paul I. Dargan - Novel and traditional club substances association to psychopathological and medical sequelae: the Ibiza project / Giovanni Martinotti, Cristina Merino del Villar, Raffaele Giorgetti, Fabrizio Schifano & Massimo Di Giannantonio - Spice drugs, synthetic cannabinoids and "spiceophrenia" / Duccio Papanti, Laura Orsolini, John M. Corkery & Fabrizio Schifano - Synthetic cannabinoids, opioids and polydrug use: clinical implications / Mariya Prilutskaya, Justin C. Yang & Andres Roman-Urrestarazu - Syntethis cathinones and related fatalities in the United Kingdom / John M. Corkery, Christine Goodair & Hugh Claridge - Marvin the Paranoid Android & Alice in Wonderland: two case reports of synthetic cathinones abuse / Pierluigi Simonato, Attilio Negri, Marco Solmi & Rita Santacroce - Clinical aspects related to methylphenidate-based NPS / Dino Lüthi & Matthias E. Liechti - The worldwide spread of "herbal highs": the case of kratom / Jessica Neicun, Darshan Singh & Eduardo Cinosi - Clinical and medical management of conditions caused by MDMA or "ecstasy" / Andrew C. Parrott - Clinical effects of 2C-B abuse / Esther Papaseit, Clara Pérez-Mañá, Débora González, Francina Fonseca, Marta Torrens & Magí Farré - "In and out of the hole": an exploration on phencyclidine derivatives / Attilio Negri & Sulaf Assi - Fentanyl and related opioids: new trends, dangers, and management / Esther Papaseit, Magí Farré, Clara Pérez-Mañá, Adriana Farré, Francina Fonseca & Marta Torrens - Designer benzodiazepines: new challenges and treatment options / Peter Maskell & Nathan E. Wilson - Misuse, recreational use and

	addiction in relation to prescription medicines / Francesco S. Bersani & Claudio Imperatori.
Other Subjects	Psychotropic Drugs--pharmacology
	Psychotropic Drugs--toxicity
	Substance-Related Disorders--prevention & control
Notes	Includes bibliographical references and index.
Additional formats	Print version: Handbook of novel psychoactive substances New York, NY: Routledge, 2019 9781138068292 (DLC) 2018026633

Handbook of novel psychoactive substances: what clinicians should know about NPS

LCCN	2018026633
Type of material	Book
Main title	Handbook of novel psychoactive substances: what clinicians should know about NPS / edited by Ornella Corazza and Andres Roman-Urrestarazu.
Published/Produced	New York, NY: Routledge, 2019.
ISBN	9781138068292 (hardback)
	9781138068308 (pbk.)
LC classification	RM315
Related names	Corazza, Ornella, editor.
	Roman-Urrestarazu, Andres, editor.
Contents	Overcoming the NPS challenge: an introduction / Ornella Corazza & Andres Roman-Urrestarazu - The need for clinical guidelines on NPS: NEPTUNE / Owen Bowden-Jones & Dima Abdulrahim - NPS: epidemiology, user group characteristics, patterns, motives and problems / Máté Kapitány-Fövény, Ariel M. Weinstein & Zsolt Demetrovics - The NPS crisis in British prisons / Shanna Marrinan, Giuseppe Bersani & Ornella Corazza - Current trends in performance and image enhancing substance use among gym goers, exercisers and athletes / Neha P. Ainsworth, Jake Shelley & Andrea Petróczi - NPS in emergency rooms: dealing with aggressiveness and psychomotor agitation / Carla Morganti, Attilio Negri, Laura Cazzaniga, Riccardo C. Gatti & Franca Davanzo - A sentinel and design model of evidence

collection on acute drug and NPS toxicity: the euroden plus project / Luke de la Rue, David M. Wood & Paul I. Dargan - Novel and traditional club substances association to psychopathological and medical sequelae: the Ibiza project / Giovanni Martinotti, Cristina Merino del Villar, Raffaele Giorgetti, Fabrizio Schifano & Massimo Di Giannantonio - Spice drugs, synthetic cannabinoids and "spiceophrenia" / Duccio Papanti, Laura Orsolini, John M. Corkery & Fabrizio Schifano - Synthetic cannabinoids, opioids and polydrug use: clinical implications / Mariya Prilutskaya, Justin C. Yang & Andres Roman-Urrestarazu - Syntethis cathinones and related fatalities in the United Kingdom / John M. Corkery, Christine Goodair & Hugh Claridge - Marvin the Paranoid Android & Alice in Wonderland: two case reports of synthetic cathinones abuse / Pierluigi Simonato, Attilio Negri, Marco Solmi & Rita Santacroce - Clinical aspects related to methylphenidate-based NPS / Dino Lüthi & Matthias E. Liechti - The worldwide spread of "herbal highs": the case of kratom / Jessica Neicun, Darshan Singh & Eduardo Cinosi - Clinical and medical management of conditions caused by MDMA or "ecstasy" / Andrew C. Parrott - Clinical effects of 2C-B abuse / Esther Papaseit, Clara Pérez-Mañá, Débora González, Francina Fonseca, Marta Torrens & Magí Farré - "In and out of the hole": an exploration on phencyclidine derivatives / Attilio Negri & Sulaf Assi - Fentanyl and related opioids: new trends, dangers, and management / Esther Papaseit, Magí Farré, Clara Pérez-Mañá, Adriana Farré, Francina Fonseca & Marta Torrens - Designer benzodiazepines: new challenges and treatment options / Peter Maskell & Nathan E. Wilson - Misuse, recreational use and addiction in relation to prescription medicines / Francesco S. Bersani & Claudio Imperatori.

Other Subjects   Psychotropic Drugs--pharmacology
Psychotropic Drugs--toxicity

	Substance-Related Disorders--prevention & control
Notes	Includes bibliographical references and index.
Additional formats	Online version: Handbook of novel psychoactive substances New York, NY: Routledge, 2019 9781315158082 (DLC) 2018027784

Herbal highs and aphrodisiacs

LCCN	2019949277
Type of material	Book
Personal name	Superweed, Mary Jane, 1975- author.
Main title	Herbal highs & aphrodisiacs / Mary Jane Superweed.
Edition	1st.
Published/Produced	Berkeley: Ronin Publishing Inc, 2019.
ISBN	9781579512859 (paperback) (ebook)
Summary	"The purpose of this book is to turn the reader on to herbs, cacti, mushrooms and other members of the vegetable kingdom which can get him high. It covers most important information, such as correct dosage, methods of use, effects, after effects and chemical nature of the psychoactive substances involved. Most of the plants mentioned are quite potent, perfectly legal and readily available either from field, forest, garden or addresses given in this book. Primarily for reasons of legal protection the author, editor and publisher of this guide do not encourage the use of any of these substances. Some of the botanicals which we discuss have potential danger. These are clearly pointed out without exaggeration. One man's treat can be another man's poison. So if any readers decide to experiment with psychedelic herbs it is best that they proceed with caution. --- excerpt from book's Introduction"-- Provided by publisher.

Key concepts in substance misuse

LCCN	2014942662
Type of material	Book
Main title	Key concepts in substance misuse / edited by Aaron Pycroft.

Published/Produced	Los Angeles: SAGE, 2015.
Description	xii, 190 pages; 21 cm.
ISBN	9781446252390 (hbk)
	1446252396 (hbk)
	9781446252406 (pbk.)
	144625240X (pbk.)
LC classification	RC564 .K78 2015
Variant title	Substance misuse
Related names	Pycroft, Aaron, editor.
Contents	Machine generated contents note: 1. Ethical Evaluations of Drug Use and Drug Policy / Aaron Pycroft - 2. The International and National Legislative Framework / Aaron Pycroft - 3. The Relationship between Politics and Scientific Knowledge in Formulating Drug Policy / Aaron Pycroft - 4. Alternatives to Prohibition / Aaron Pycroft - 5. Sedatives / Aaron Pycroft - 6. Stimulants / Aaron Pycroft - 7. Opiates / Aaron Pycroft - 8. Hallucinogens / Aaron Pycroft - 9. Drugs with Mixed Effects / Aaron Pycroft - 10. Poly Drug Use / Aaron Pycroft - 11. New Psychoactive Substances (Legal Highs) / Aaron Pycroft - 12. Addiction as a Complex Adaptive System / Aaron Pycroft - 13. The Evolutionary Context / Aaron Pycroft - 14. Dependence Syndromes / Aaron Pycroft - 15. Psychological Perspectives / Aaron Pycroft - 16. Dual Diagnosis and the Context of Exclusion / Aaron Pycroft - 17. Harm Reduction / Anita Green - 18. The Concept of Recovery / Tony Shea - 19. The Purposes and Methods of Detoxification from Illicit Drugs / Tim Leighton - 20. The Purposes and Methods of Detoxification from Alcohol / Rebecca Lee - 21. The Major Talking Therapies / Ann Spooner / Pamela Campbell - 22. Buddhism and Addiction / Trevor Smith - 23. Criminal Justice Interventions / Devin Ashwood - 24. Evidence-based Practice, Research and Outcome Monitoring / Bernie Heath - 25. The Core Skills in Working with Substance Misuse / Jane

	Winston - 26. Whole Systems Approaches / Angela Woods.
LC Subjects	Substance abuse.
	Drug abuse.
	Drug addiction.
Other Subjects	Substance-Related Disorders.
	Drug Users--Psychology.
	Psychotropic Drugs.
	Drug and Narcotic Control.
	Drug abuse.
	Drug addiction.
	Substance abuse.
Notes	Includes bibliographical references and index.
Series	SAGE key concepts
	SAGE key concepts.

Killer high: a history of war in six drugs

LCCN	2019005585
Type of material	Book
Personal name	Andreas, Peter, 1965- author.
Main title	Killer high: a history of war in six drugs / Peter Andreas.
Published/Produced	New York, NY: Oxford University Press, [2020]
Description	ix, 338 pages: illustrations; 25 cm
ISBN	9780190463014 (hardback)
LC classification	RC971.A53 2020
Portion of title	History of war in six drugs
Summary	" There is growing alarm over how drugs increasingly empower terrorists, insurgents, traffickers, and gangs. But by looking back not just years and decades but centuries, Peter Andreas reveals that the drugs-conflict nexus is actually an old story, and that powerful states have been its biggest beneficiaries. In his path-breaking Killer High, Andreas shows how six psychoactive drugs--ranging from old to relatively new, mild to potent, licit to illicit, natural to synthetic--have proven to be particularly important war ingredients. This sweeping history tells the story of war from antiquity to the modern age through the

lens of alcohol, tobacco, caffeine, opium, amphetamines, and cocaine. Beer and wine drenched ancient and medieval battlefields, and the distilling revolution lubricated the conquest and ethnic cleansing of the New World. Tobacco became globalized through soldiering, with soldiers hooked on smoking and governments hooked on taxing it. Caffeine and opium fueled imperial expansion and warfare. The commercialization of amphetamines in the twentieth century energized soldiers to fight harder, longer, and faster, while cocaine stimulated an increasingly militarized drug war that produced casualty numbers surpassing most civil wars. As Andreas demonstrates, armed conflict has become progressively more "drugged" with the introduction, mass production, and global spread of mind-altering substances. As a result, we cannot understand the history of war without including drugs, and we similarly cannot understand the history of drugs without including war. From ancient brews and battles to meth and modern warfare, drugs and war have grown up together and become addicted to each other. "-- Provided by publisher.

"In his path-breaking Killer High, Andreas shows how six psychoactive drugs--ranging from old to relatively new, mild to potent, licit to illicit, natural to synthetic--have proven to be particularly important war ingredients. This sweeping history tells the story of war from antiquity to the modern age through the lens of alcohol, tobacco, caffeine, opium, amphetamines, and cocaine. Beer and wine drenched ancient and medieval battlefields, and the distilling revolution lubricated the conquest and ethnic cleansing of the New World. Tobacco became globalized through soldiering, with soldiers hooked on smoking and governments hooked on taxing it. Caffeine and opium fueled imperial expansion and warfare. The commercialization of amphetamines in the twentieth century energized soldiers to fight harder, longer, and faster, while cocaine stimulated an increasingly militarized drug war that produced casualty numbers surpassing most civil wars. As Andreas demonstrates, armed conflict has become progressively more "drugged" with the introduction, mass production, and global spread of mind-altering substances. As a result, we cannot understand the history of war without including drugs, and we similarly cannot understand the history of drugs without including war. From ancient brews and battles to meth and modern warfare, drugs and war have grown up together and become addicted to each other"-- Provided by publisher.

LC Subjects	Medicine, Military--History--Miscellanea.
	Soldiers--Drug use--History.
	Soldiers--Substance use--History.
	Drug utilization--History.
	Drug abuse--History.
	Military art and science--Miscellanea.
	Military history--Miscellanea.
Other Subjects	History / Military / General.
Notes	Includes bibliographical references (pages 269-316) and index.

Legalizing cannabis: experiences, lessons and scenarios

LCCN	2019048744
Type of material	Book
Main title	Legalizing cannabis: experiences, lessons and scenarios / Tom Decorte, Simon Lenton, Chris Wilkins.
Published/Produced	Abingdon, Oxon; New York, NY: Routledge, 2020.
ISBN	9781138370906 (hardback)
	(ebook)
LC classification	K3641.L44 2020
Related names	Decorte, Tom, editor.
	Lenton, Simon, 1961- editor.
	Wilkins, Chris, editor.
Summary	"The book explores how we should evaluate the models of cannabis legalization as they have been

implemented in several jurisdictions in the past few years; the specific models for future cannabis legalization that have been developed and how similar or different they are they from the models already implemented; as well as the lessons that can be drawn from attempts to regulate other psychoactive substances, such as alcohol, tobacco, pharmaceuticals and "legal highs", and other "vice" activities such as gambling and prostitution"-- Provided by publisher.

Contents Introduction: the coming cannabis revolution / Tom Decorte, Simon Lenton and Chris Wilkins - The uneven repeal of cannabis prohibition in the United States / Bryce Pardo - Practical lessons learned from the first years of the regulated recreational cannabis market in Colorado / Todd Subritzky, Simon Lenton, Simone Pettigrew - Recreational marijuana legalization in Washington State: benefits and harms / Clayton Mosher and Scott Akins - A century of cannabis control in Canada: a brief overview of history, context and policy frameworks from prohibition to legalization / Benedikt Fischer, Cayley Russell, Neil Boyd - Uruguay: the first country to legalize cannabis / Rosario Queirolo - Cannabis decriminalization policies across the globe / Niamh Eastwood - "More than just counting the plants": different home cannabis cultivation policies, cannabis supply contexts and approaches to their evaluation / Vendula Belackova, Katinka van de Ven, Michaela Roubalova (Stefunkova) - City-level policies of regulating recreational cannabis in Europe: from pilot projects to "local customization"? / Tom Blickman & Catherine Sandwell - Lessons learned from the alcohol regulation perspective / Tim Stockwell, Norman Giesbrecht, Adam Sherk, Gerald Thomas, Kate Vallance and Ashley Wettlaufer - Lessons from tobacco regulation for cannabis product regulation / Coral Gartner & Wayne Hall - How not to legalize cannabis: lessons from New Zealand's experiment with regulating "legal highs" / Marta Rychert - Coffeeshops in the Netherlands: regulating the front door and the back door / Dirk J. Korf - Cannabis social clubs in Spain: recent legal developments / Xabier Arana and Òscar Parés - Swiss cannabis policies / Simon Anderfuhren-Biget, Frank Zobel, Cédric Heeb, Jean-Félix Savary - The Australian experience and opportunities for cannabis law reform / Caitlin Elizabeth Hughes - Cannabis policy reform: the Jamaica's experience / Vicki J. Hanson - The risks of cannabis industry funding of community and drug treatment services: insights from gambling / Chris Wilkins, Marta Rychert - Insights for the design of Cannabis Social Club regulation / Tom Decorte, Mafalda Pardal - Conclusion / Chris Wilkins, Simon Lenton and Tom Decorte.

LC Subjects	Drug legalization.
	Cannabis--Law and legislation
	Marijuana industry--Law and legislation
Notes	Includes bibliographical references and index.
Series	Routledge studies in crime and society

Mental health in prisons: critical perspectives on treatment and confinement

LCCN	2019762678
Type of material	Book
Main title	Mental Health in Prisons: Critical Perspectives on Treatment and Confinement / edited by Alice Mills, Kathleen Kendall.
Edition	1st ed. 2018.
Published/Produced	Cham: Springer International Publishing: Imprint: Palgrave Macmillan, 2018.
Description	1 online resource (XXIII, 385 pages 7 illustrations) PDF
ISBN	9783319940908
Related names	Kendall, Kathleen, editor.
	Mills, Alice, editor.

Summary This book examines how the prison environment, architecture and culture can affect mental health as well as determine both the type and delivery of mental health services. It also discusses how non-medical practices, such as peer support and prison education programs, offer the possibility of transformative practice and support. By drawing on international contributions, it furthermore demonstrates how mental health in prisons is affected by wider socio-economic and cultural factors, and how in recent years neo-liberalism has abandoned, criminalised and contained large numbers of the world's most marginalised and vulnerable populations. Overall, this collection challenges the dominant narrative of individualism by focusing instead on the relationship between structural inequalities, suffering, survival and punishment. Chapter 2 is available open access under a Creative Commons Attribution 4.0 International License via link.springer.com.

Contents Chapter 1. Introduction - PART 1. Penal Power and the Psy Disciplines: Contextualising Mental Health and Imprisonment - Chapter 2. 'We Are Recreating Bedlam': A History of Mental Illness and Prison Systems in England and Ireland; Catherine Cox and Hilary Marland - Chapter 3. The Architecture of Psychiatry and the Architecture of Incarceration; Simon Cross and Yvonne Jewkes - Chapter 4. Psychological Jurisprudence and the Relational Problems of De-vitalization and Finalization: Revisiting the Society of Captives Thesis; Bruce A. Arrigo and Brian G. Sellers - PART 2. Care versus Custody - Chapter 5. Care versus Custody: Challenges in the Provision of Prison Mental Healthcare; Alice Mills and Kathleen Kendall - Chapter 6. How do New Psychoactive Substances Affect the Mental Health of Prisoners?; Hattie Moyes - Chapter 7. 'There was no understanding, there was no care, there was no looking after me': The impact

	of the prison environment on the mental health of female prisoners; Anastasia Jablonska and Rosie Meek - PART 3. Dividing Practices: Structural Violence, Mental health and Imprisonment - Chapter 8. Institutions of Default and Management: Aboriginal Women with Mental and Cognitive Disability in Prison; Ruth McCausland, Elizabeth McEntyre and Eileen Baldry - Chapter 9. Culture, Mental Illness, and Prison: A New Zealand Perspective; James Cavney and Susan Hatters Friedman - Chapter10. 'Malignant Reality': Mental Ill-Health and Self-Inflicted Deaths in England and Wales; Joe Sim - Chapter 11. Institutional Captives: US Women Trapped in the Medical / Correctional / Welfare Circuit; Maureen Norton-Hawk and Susan Sered - Chapter 12. Queer and Trans Incarceration Distress: Considerations from a Mad Queer Abolitionist Perspective; Andrea Daley and Kim Radford - PART 3. Alternative Penal Practices and Communities - Chapter 13. A Sense of Belonging: The Walls to Bridges Educational Program as a Healing Space; Shoshana Pollack and Denise Edwards - Chapter 14. Coping with incarceration: The emerging case for the utility of peer-support programs in prison; Christian Perrin - Chapter 15. Conclusion; Kathleen Kendall and Alice Mills.
LC Subjects	Corrections. Criminology. Critical Psychology. Forensic Psychology. Human rights. Punishment. Sex and law.
Other Subjects	Prison and Punishment. Critical Psychology. Forensic Psychology. Gender, Sexuality and Law. Human Rights and Crime.

Additional formats	Print version: Mental health in prisons. 9783319940892 (DLC) 2018946175
	Printed edition: 9783030405083
	Printed edition: 9783319940892
	Printed edition: 9783319940915
Series	Palgrave Studies in Prisons and Penology
	Palgrave Studies in Prisons and Penology

My psychedelic explorations: the healing power and transformational potential of psychoactive substances

LCCN	2020002914
Type of material	Book
Personal name	Naranjo, Claudio, author.
Uniform title	Exploraciones psicodélicas. English
Main title	My psychedelic explorations: the healing power and transformational potential of psychoactive substances / Claudio Naranjo, M.D.; translated by Tania Mollart Rogerson.
Published/Produced	Rochester, Vermont: Park Street Press, 2020.
Description	xviii, 430 pages: illustrations; 23 cm
ISBN	9781644110584 (paperback)
	(ebook)
LC classification	RM324.8.N3713 2020
Related names	Mollart Rogerson, Tania, translator.
Summary	"Claudio Naranjo's psychedelic autobiography with previously unpublished interviews and research papers. Explores Dr. Naranjo's pioneering work with MDMA, ayahuasca, cannabis, iboga, and psilocybin. Shares his personal accounts of psychedelic sessions and experimentation, including his work with Alexander Sasha Shulgin and Leo Zeff. Includes the author's reflections on the spiritual aspects of psychedelics and his recommended techniques for controlled induction of altered states"-- Provided by publisher.
LC Subjects	Hallucinogenic drugs--Therapeutic use.
	Psychopharmacology.
	Spiritual life.
	Psychotherapy.

Notes	Includes bibliographical references and index.
Additional formats	Online version: Naranjo, Claudio, My psychedelic explorations First U.S. edition. Rochester: Park Street Press, 2020. 9781644110591 (DLC) 2020002915

My psychedelic explorations: the healing power and transformational potential of psychoactive substances

LCCN	2020002915
Type of material	Book
Personal name	Naranjo, Claudio, author.
Uniform title	Exploraciones psicodélicas. English
Main title	My psychedelic explorations: the healing power and transformational potential of psychoactive substances / Claudio Naranjo, M.D.; translated by Tania Mollart Rogerson.
Edition	First U.S. edition.
Published/Produced	Rochester: Park Street Press, 2020.
Description	1 online resource
ISBN	9781644110591 (ebook)
	(paperback)
LC classification	RM324.8
Related names	Mollart Rogerson, Tania, translator.
Summary	"Claudio Naranjo's psychedelic autobiography with previously unpublished interviews and research papers. Explores Dr. Naranjo's pioneering work with MDMA, ayahuasca, cannabis, iboga, and psilocybin. Shares his personal accounts of psychedelic sessions and experimentation, including his work with Alexander Sasha Shulgin and Leo Zeff. Includes the author's reflections on the spiritual aspects of psychedelics and his recommended techniques for controlled induction of altered states"-- Provided by publisher.
LC Subjects	Hallucinogenic drugs--Therapeutic use.
	Psychopharmacology.
	Spiritual life.
	Psychotherapy.
Notes	Includes bibliographical references and index.

Additional formats	Print version: Naranjo, Claudio. My psychedelic explorations First U.S. edition. Rochester: Park Street Press, 2020. 9781644110584 (DLC) 2020002914

Neuropharmacology of new psychoactive substances (NPS): the science behind the headlines

LCCN	2017937529
Type of material	Book
Personal name	Baumann, Michael H.
Main title	Neuropharmacology of new psychoactive substances (NPS): the science behind the headlines / Michael H. Baumann.
Edition	1st edition.
Published/Produced	New York, NY: Springer Berlin Heidelberg, 2017.
ISBN	9783319524429 (alk. paper)

Neuropharmacology of New Psychoactive Substances (NPS): the Science Behind the Headlines

LCCN	2019750434
Type of material	Book
Main title	Neuropharmacology of New Psychoactive Substances (NPS): The Science Behind the Headlines / edited by Michael H. Baumann, Richard A. Glennon, Jenny L. Wiley.
Edition	1st ed. 2017.
Published/Produced	Cham: Springer International Publishing: Imprint: Springer, 2017.
Description	1 online resource (VIII, 380 pages 81 illustrations, 13 illustrations in color.) PDF
ISBN	9783319524443
Related names	Baumann, Michael H. editor. Glennon, Richard A. editor. Wiley, Jenny L. editor.
Summary	Designer drugs, or new psychoactive substances (NPS), are synthetic chemicals that mimic the effects of classic drugs of abuse. There has been an alarming worldwide increase in the abuse of NPS in recent years. NPS are cheap, easy to obtain, and often

	legally available. In this volume, leading experts summarize the latest studies regarding the molecular mechanisms of action, behavioral effects, and adverse consequences of popular NPS. Specific chapters clarify the differences between various types of NPS, namely: stimulants, cannabinoids and hallucinogens. Thus, this volume broadens our understanding of NPS and provides insight into the rapidly evolving "new drug" phenomenon.
LC Subjects	Neurosciences.
	Pharmacology.
	Psychopharmacology.
	Public health.
Other Subjects	Neurosciences.
	Pharmacology/Toxicology.
	Psychopharmacology.
	Public Health.
Additional formats	Print version: Neuropharmacology of new psychoactive substances (NPS): the science behind the headlines 9783319524429 (DLC) 2017937529
	Printed edition: 9783319524429
	Printed edition: 9783319524436
	Printed edition: 9783319849065
Series	Current Topics in Behavioral Neurosciences, 1866-3370; 32
	Current Topics in Behavioral Neurosciences, 1866-3370; 32

Neurotheology: how science can enlighten us about spirituality

LCCN	2017044209
Type of material	Book
Personal name	Newberg, Andrew B., 1966- author.
Main title	Neurotheology: how science can enlighten us about spirituality / Andrew Newberg.
Published/Produced	New York: Columbia University Press, [2018]
Description	vi, 321 pages: illustrations; 24 cm
ISBN	9780231179041 (hardback)
LC classification	QP355.2 .N57 2018

Bibliography

Summary   "With the advent of the modern cognitive neurosciences, along with anthropological and historical research, the scientific study of religious and spiritual phenomena has become far more sophisticated and wide-ranging. It suggests answers as to how and why religion became so prominent in human societies and in human consciousness. Neurotheology--a term coined by Aldous Huxley in 1962 in his novel Island and introduced into the scientific literature in the 1990s by Newberg and others--explores some of the most controversial positions including the argument that religion was a necessary condition of cohesive societies, morality, and a sense of purpose. The book considers brain development from an evolutionary perspective and assesses how religious and spiritual beliefs and experiences arose and whether such evolutionary evidence eliminates the need for a religious explanation. Newberg demonstrates that religious beliefs and emotions can be both beneficial and detrimental in people's lives. For some, religion provides a means toward compassion, openness, and understanding; others turn to highly destructive acts, as is the case with suicide bombers. What is happening in the brains of such people? Are they pathological? And what of practices such as meditation, prayer, and the ingestion of psychoactive substances? Neuroimaging studies can show how these practices affect people in the moment and over a lifetime. Finally, the book investigates the deeper implications of a neurotheological approach. Does the neuroscientific study of religion negate any or all of the truth claims of religion? How does neurotheology address the "big questions" such as: What is the meaning of life? Why are we here? And what is the true nature of reality?"-- Provided by publisher.

LC Subjects   Neurophysiology--Religious aspects.
Brain--Religious aspects.

	Spirituality.
	Psychology, Religious.
Notes	Includes bibliographical references (pages 289-314) and index.
Additional formats	Online version: Newberg, Andrew B., 1966- author. Neurotheology New York: Columbia University Press, [2018] 9780231546775 (DLC) 2017052056

New psychoactive substances: pharmacology, clinical, forensic and analytical toxicology

LCCN	2018966537
Type of material	Book
Main title	New psychoactive substances: pharmacology, clinical, forensic and analytical toxicology / [edited by] Hans H. Maurer.
Published/Produced	New York, NY: Springer Berlin Heidelberg, 2019.
ISBN	9783030105600 (alk. paper)

New psychoactive substances: pharmacology, clinical, forensic and analytical toxicology

LCCN	2019768225
Type of material	Book
Main title	New Psychoactive Substances: Pharmacology, Clinical, Forensic and Analytical Toxicology / edited by Hans H. Maurer, Simon D. Brandt.
Edition	1st ed. 2018.
Published/Produced	Cham: Springer International Publishing: Imprint: Springer, 2018.
Description	1 online resource (X, 566 pages 90 illustrations, 28 illustrations in color.)
	PDF
ISBN	9783030105617
Related names	Brandt, Simon D, editor.
	Maurer, Hans H, editor.
Summary	This volume is designed to feature the pharmacology of new psychoactive substances, legislative aspects, information exchange including epidemiology, and clinical, forensic, and analytical toxicology in order

	to facilitate the understanding of this complex and rapidly developing phenomenon.
Contents	Preface - Part I General Aspects - 1. Self-Experiments with Psychoactive Substances: A Historical Perspective - 2. Responding to New Psychoactive Substances in the European Union: Early Warning, Risk Assessment, and Control Measures - 3. Emergence, Diversity, and Control of New Psychoactive Substances: A Global Perspective - 4. Epidemiology of NPS Based Confirmed Overdose Cases: The STRIDA Project - Part II Drug Classes - 5. Neuropharmacology of Synthetic Cathinones - 6. Pharmacology of MDMA- and Amphetamine-Like New Psychoactive Substances - 7. The Chemistry and Pharmacology of Synthetic Cannabinoid Receptor Agonists as New Psychoactive Substances: Origins - 8. Molecular pharmacology of synthetic cannabinoids: Evolution - 9. Synthetic Opioids - 10. Designer Benzodiazepines: Another Class of New Psychoactive Substances - 11. Serotonergic Psychedelics: Experimental Approaches for Assessing Mechanisms of Action - 12. 1,2-Diarylethylamine- and Ketamine-Based New Psychoactive Substances - 13. Phencyclidine-Based New Psychoactive Substances - Part III Clinical, Forensic, and Analytical Toxicology - 14. Bioanalytical Methods for New Psychoactive Substances - 15. Wastewater Analysis for Community-Wide Drugs Use Assessment - 16. Toxicokinetics of NPS: Update 2017 - 17. Patterns of Acute Toxicity Associated with New Psychoactive Substances - 18. Fatal Poisonings Associated with New Psychoactive Substances.
LC Subjects	Pharmacology.
Other Subjects	Pharmacology/Toxicology.
Additional formats	Print version: New psychoactive substances: pharmacology, clinical, forensic and analytical toxicology 9783030105600 (DLC) 2018966537 Printed edition: 9783030105600

	Printed edition: 9783030105624
Series	Handbook of Experimental Pharmacology, 0171-2004; 252
	Handbook of Experimental Pharmacology, 0171-2004; 252

New psychoactive substances in South Korea: recent trends monitored by the National Forensic Service during 2009-2016.

LCCN	2018492735
Type of material	Book
Uniform title	Sinjong mayangnyu yuhyŏng punsŏk. English.
Main title	New psychoactive substances in South Korea: recent trends monitored by the National Forensic Service during 2009-2016.
Published/Produced	Wonju-si, Gangwon-do: National Forensic Service, 2017.
Description	55 pages: color illustrations; 26 cm
ISBN	9788995715253
LC classification	RM315.S53513 2017
Related names	Kungnip Kwahak Susa Yŏn'guwŏn (Korea), issuing body.
LC Subjects	Psychotropic drugs--Korea (South)--History--21st century.
	Designer drugs--Korea (South)--History--21st century.
	Drug abuse--Government policy--Korea (South)
Notes	Palgan tŭngnok pŏnho: 11-1740153-000006-01.

Novel psychoactive substances: classification, pharmacology and toxicology

LCCN	2021940475
Type of material	Book
Main title	Novel psychoactive substances: classification, pharmacology and toxicology / Paul I. Dargan, David M. Wood.
Edition	2.
Published/Produced	San Diego: Academic Press is an imprint of Elsevier, 2021.
ISBN	9780128187883 (hardback)

Related names	Dargan, Paul I., editor.
	Wood, David M., editor.
Summary	"Novel Psychoactive Substances: Classification, Pharmacology and Toxicology, Second Edition provides readers with a comprehensive examination on the classification, detection, supply and availability of novel psychoactive substances, otherwise known as "legal highs." The book covers individual classes of novel psychoactive substances that have recently emerged onto the recreational drug scene and provides an overview of the pharmacology of the substance and a discussion of their associated acute and chronic harm and toxicity. This second edition addresses drugs new to the scene, with completely updated and revised chapters. Written by international experts in the field, this multi-authored book is an essential reference for scientists, clinicians, academics, and regulatory and law enforcement professionals"-- Provided by publisher.

Novel psychoactive substances: policy, economics and drug regulation

LCCN	2019770340
Type of material	Book
Main title	Novel Psychoactive Substances: Policy, Economics and Drug Regulation / edited by Ornella Corazza, Andres Roman-Urrestarazu.
Edition	1st ed. 2017.
Published/Produced	Cham: Springer International Publishing: Imprint: Springer, 2017.
Description	1 online resource (XXII, 178 pages 8 illustrations, 6 illustrations in color.)
	PDF
ISBN	9783319606002
Related names	Corazza, Ornella, editor.
	Roman-Urrestarazu, Andres, editor.
Summary	In light of the recent emergence of New Psychoactive Substances (NPS) on a global scale, this book provides a timely analysis of the social and economic impact of the NPS phenomenon, and of the global

	policy and regulatory responses to it. It presents the first comprehensive overview of the international regulation, policy and market structure of the NPS phenomenon, offering a guide to inform legislative discussions and demonstrating from a comparative perspective the different approaches used to address the rise of NPS to date. It covers topics such as organized crime, drug markets, clinical evidence on NPS, and different regulatory measures. Overall, this highly informative and well-structured repository of different experiences with NPS policy, law and regulation offers an essential primary source of evidence for anyone interested in the area of drug and NPS policy, health economics and public health.
Contents	1. The Global Emergence of NPS: An Analysis of a New Drug Trend - 2. Legislating NPS in the European Union - 3. Regulation as Global Drug Governance - How New is the NPS Phenomenon? - 4. Anti-Doping Challenges with Novel Psychoactive Substances in Sport - 5. Exploring Novel Policy Responses to NPS and 'legal highs' in New Zealand, Poland, Republic of Ireland and the United Kingdom - 6. Regulating NPS in the Middle East: A Critical Juncture - 7. Finding Novel Policy Response to the Challenge of NPS in Kazakhstan: Reconsidering Existing Policy and the Work of Health Professionals - 8. NPS Policy Pitfalls: The Implementation and Management Challenges Within the Prison, Police and Health Services in the United Kingdom - 9. NPS: An Opportunity to Move From Blanket Prohibition to a More Functionalist Approach? - 10. The Challenges in Interpreting National-Level Strategic Indicators: A Drug Enforcement Administration Analyst's Perspective - 11. Harmonizing NPS Legislation Across the European Union: An Utopia? - 12. New psychoactive substances: The Regulatory Experience and Assessment of Options.
LC Subjects	Health care management. Health economics.

Other Subjects	Health services administration. Pharmacy. Public health. Health Economics. Health Care Management. Pharmacy. Public Health.
Additional formats	Print version: Novel psychoactive substances 9783319605999 (DLC) 2017947704 Printed edition: 9783319605999 Printed edition: 9783319606019 Printed edition: 9783319868967

Novel psychoactive substances

LCCN	2017947704
Type of material	Book
Main title	Novel psychoactive substances / [edited by] Ornella Corazza.
Published/Produced	New York, NY: Springer Berlin Heidelberg, 2017.
ISBN	9783319605999 (alk. paper)

Prohibitions and psychoactive substances in history, culture and theory

LCCN	2019980843
Type of material	Book
Main title	Prohibitions and psychoactive substances in history, culture and theory / edited by Susannah Wilson.
Published/Produced	New York: Routledge/Taylor & Francis Group, 2019.
Description	1 online resource.
ISBN	9780429289729 (ebk) 9781000011951 (epub) 9780415015486 (epub) 9780415015202 (pdf) 9780415015349 (mobi) (hbk: alk. paper)
LC classification	RM315
Related names	Wilson, Susannah, 1976- editor.
LC Subjects	Psychotropic drugs. Prohibition.
Notes	Includes bibliographical references and index.

Additional formats	Print version: Prohibitions and psychoactive substances in history, culture and theory New York: Routledge/Taylor & Francis Group, 2019. 9780367257637 (hbk: alk. paper) (DLC) 2019013719
Series	Warwick series in the humanities

Prohibitions and psychoactive substances in history, culture and theory

LCCN	2019013719
Type of material	Book
Main title	Prohibitions and psychoactive substances in history, culture and theory / edited by Susannah Wilson.
Published/Produced	New York, NY: Routledge, 2019.
ISBN	9780367257637 (hbk: alk. paper)
LC classification	RM315.P7154 2019
Related names	Wilson, Susannah, 1976- editor.
LC Subjects	Psychotropic drugs. Prohibition.
Notes	Includes bibliographical references and index.
Additional formats	Online version: Prohibitions and psychoactive substances in history, culture and theory. New York, NY: Routledge, 2019. 9780429289729 (DLC) 2019980843
Series	Warwick series in the humanities

Psychobiological issues in substance use and misuse

LCCN	2020038194
Type of material	Book
Main title	Psychobiological issues in substance use and misuse / edited by Philip N. Murphy.
Published/Produced	London; New York: Routledge, Taylor & Francis Group, 2021.
Description	1 online resource.
ISBN	9780429296345 (ebook) (hardback) (paperback)
LC classification	HV4998
Related names	Murphy, Philip N., editor.

Summary	"In this book, Murphy brings together a team of international experts to review cutting-edge scientific literature from the field of psychobiology which addresses important questions and broadens our understanding of substance use behaviours. The reader is introduced to the multi-faceted nature of substance use and misuse, and its growing need to be discussed across diverse disciplines and perspectives. The book also addresses important questions regarding public policy and professional practice in the context of different social and cultural environments, and comments on the methodological and ethical approach in substance use and misuse. Chapters explore a spectrum of substances, which include: cocaine, alcohol, ecstasy (MDMA), methamphetamine, synthetic cannabinoids, tobacco, ketamine, novel psychoactive substances, and vaping products. The use of these substances poses important questions for science and for society. This book is written to help academics, practitioners, and students in a variety of academic and professional disciplines answer those questions while staying up to date with the psychobiological literature. This is a vital resource for professionals and upper-level undergraduate and postgraduate students undertaking research in areas related to biological Psychology, biology, health studies, and medicine"-- Provided by publisher.
LC Subjects	Substance abuse--Psychological aspects. Substance abuse--Prevention. Substance abuse--Treatment. Drug abuse--Prevention. Drug abuse--Treatment.
Notes	Includes bibliographical references and index.
Additional formats	Print version: Psychobiological issues in substance use and misuse 1 Edition. New York: Routledge, 2021. 9780367273606 (DLC) 2020038193
Series	Current issues in psychobiology

Psychobiological issues in substance use and misuse

LCCN	2020038193
Type of material	Book
Main title	Psychobiological issues in substance use and misuse / edited by Philip N. Murphy.
Edition	1 Edition.
Published/Produced	New York: Routledge, 2021.
ISBN	9780367273606 (hardback)
	9780367273613 (paperback)
	(ebook)
LC classification	HV4998.P793 2021
Related names	Murphy, Philip N., editor.
Summary	"In this book, Murphy brings together a team of international experts to review cutting-edge scientific literature from the field of psychobiology which addresses important questions and broadens our understanding of substance use behaviours. The reader is introduced to the multi-faceted nature of substance use and misuse, and its growing need to be discussed across diverse disciplines and perspectives. The book also addresses important questions regarding public policy and professional practice in the context of different social and cultural environments, and comments on the methodological and ethical approach in substance use and misuse. Chapters explore a spectrum of substances, which include: cocaine, alcohol, ecstasy (MDMA), methamphetamine, synthetic cannabinoids, tobacco, ketamine, novel psychoactive substances, and vaping products. The use of these substances poses important questions for science and for society. This book is written to help academics, practitioners, and students in a variety of academic and professional disciplines answer those questions while staying up to date with the psychobiological literature. This is a vital resource for professionals and upper-level undergraduate and postgraduate students undertaking research in areas related to biological Psychology,

LC Subjects	biology, health studies, and medicine"-- Provided by publisher. Substance abuse--Psychological aspects. Substance abuse--Prevention. Substance abuse--Treatment. Drug abuse--Prevention. Drug abuse--Treatment.
Notes	Includes bibliographical references and index.
Additional formats	Online version: Psychobiological issues in substance use and misuse 1. New York: Routledge, 2021. 9780429296345 (DLC) 2020038194
Series	Current issues in psychobiology

Quick fixes: drugs in America from prohibition to the 21st-century binge

LCCN	2022058907
Type of material	Book
Personal name	Fong, Benjamin Y., author.
Main title	Quick fixes: drugs in America from Prohibition to the 21st-century binge / Benjamin Y. Fong.
Published/Produced	London; New York: Verso, 2023.
ISBN	9781804290170 (hardback) (ebook)
LC classification	HV5825.F65 2023
Summary	"Fong examines Americans' fraught relationship with psychoactive substances"-- Provided by publisher.
Contents	Introduction - Coffee, or the Serene Delight - Cigarettes, or Knowledge Is Not Power - Alcohol, or Commodity Fetishism - Opiates, or Civilizing the Orient - Amphetamines, or Inappropriate Perseverance - Psychotropics, or Diagnostic Creeps and Rational Paranoids - Psychedelics, or the Dialectic of Control - Addendum on Peyote - Addendum on Dissociative Anesthetics - Cocaine, or Hyperreality - Marijuana, or Profit Wins in the End - Conclusion.
LC Subjects	Drug abuse--United States--History. Drugs of abuse--United States--History. Psychotropic drugs--United States--History.
Notes	Includes bibliographical references.

Additional formats	Online version: Fong, Benjamin Y. Quick fixes London; New York: Verso, 2023 9781804290200 (DLC) 2022058908
Series	The Jacobin series

Religious freedom and the global regulation of ayahuasca

LCCN	2022044241
Type of material	Book
Main title	Religious freedom and the global regulation of ayahuasca / edited by Beatriz Labate and Clancy Cavnar.
Published/Produced	Milton Park, Abingdon, Oxon; New York, NY: Routledge, 2023.
ISBN	9780367028756 (hardback)
	9781032439327 (paperback)
	(ebook)
LC classification	BF209.A93 R45 2023
Related names	Labate, Beatriz Caiuby, editor.
	Cavnar, Clancy, editor.
Summary	"This book offers a comprehensive view of the legal, political, and ethical challenges related to the global regulation of ayahuasca, bringing together an international and interdisciplinary group of scholars. Ayahuasca is a psychoactive brew containing DMT, which is a Schedule I substance under the United Nations Convention on Psychotropic Substances, and the legality of its ritual use has been interpreted differently throughout the world. The chapters in this volume reflect on the complex implications of the international expansion of ayahuasca, from health, spirituality, and human rights impacts on individuals, to legal and policy impacts on national governments. While freedom of religion is generally protected, this protection depends on the recognition of a religion's legitimacy, and whether particular practices may be deemed a threat to public health, safety or morality. Through a comparative analysis of different contexts in North America, South America and Europe in which ayahuasca is consumed, the book investigates

Bibliography

LC Subjects	Ayahuasca--Physiological effect.
	Ayahuasca--Law and legislation.
	Hallucinogenic drugs and religious experience.
	Freedom of religion.
Notes	Includes bibliographical references and index.
Additional formats	Online version: Religious freedom and the global regulation of ayahuasca Milton Park, Abingdon, Oxon; New York, NY: Routledge, 2023 9780429001161 (DLC) 2022044242

the conceptual, philosophical, and legal distinctions among the fields of shamanism, religion, and medicine. It will be particularly relevant to scholars with an interest in Indigenous religion and in religion and law"-- Provided by publisher.

Religious freedom and the global regulation of ayahuasca

LCCN	2022044242
Type of material	Book
Main title	Religious freedom and the global regulation of ayahuasca / edited by Beatriz Labate and Clancy Cavnar.
Published/Produced	Milton Park, Abingdon, Oxon; New York, NY: Routledge, 2023.
Description	1 online resource
ISBN	9780429001161 (ebook)
	(hardback)
	(paperback)
LC classification	BF209.A93
Related names	Labate, Beatriz Caiuby, editor.
	Cavnar, Clancy, editor.
Summary	"This book offers a comprehensive view of the legal, political, and ethical challenges related to the global regulation of ayahuasca, bringing together an international and interdisciplinary group of scholars. Ayahuasca is a psychoactive brew containing DMT, which is a Schedule I substance under the United Nations Convention on Psychotropic Substances, and the legality of its ritual use has been interpreted differently throughout the world. The chapters in this

	volume reflect on the complex implications of the international expansion of ayahuasca, from health, spirituality, and human rights impacts on individuals, to legal and policy impacts on national governments. While freedom of religion is generally protected, this protection depends on the recognition of a religion's legitimacy, and whether particular practices may be deemed a threat to public health, safety or morality. Through a comparative analysis of different contexts in North America, South America and Europe in which ayahuasca is consumed, the book investigates the conceptual, philosophical, and legal distinctions among the fields of shamanism, religion, and medicine. It will be particularly relevant to scholars with an interest in Indigenous religion and in religion and law"-- Provided by publisher.
LC Subjects	Ayahuasca--Physiological effect.
	Ayahuasca--Law and legislation.
	Hallucinogenic drugs and religious experience.
	Freedom of religion.
Notes	Includes bibliographical references and index.
Additional formats	Print version: Religious freedom and the global regulation of ayahuasca Milton Park, Abingdon, Oxon; New York, NY: Routledge, 2023 9780367028756 (DLC) 2022044241

Seeking the sacred with psychoactive substances: chemical paths to spirituality and to God

LCCN	2014021610
Type of material	Book
Main title	Seeking the sacred with psychoactive substances: chemical paths to spirituality and to God / J. Harold Ellens, editor; foreword by The Rev. Dr. Alexander Riegel.
Published/Produced	Santa Barbara: Praeger, 2014-
Description	volumes; 25 cm.
ISBN	9781440830877 (alk. paper)
LC classification	BL65.D7 S44 2014
Related names	Ellens, J. Harold, 1932- editor.

Contents	Volume 1. History and practices - v. 2. Insights, arguments, and controversies
LC Subjects	Hallucinogenic drugs and religious experience. Psychology and religion. Psychotropic drugs. Spiritual life. Spirituality.
Notes	Includes index.
Series	Psychology, religion, and spirituality

Substance use and abuse: everything matters

LCCN	2016438695
Type of material	Book
Personal name	Csiernik, Rick, author.
Main title	Substance use and abuse: everything matters / Rick Csiernik.
Edition	Second edition.
Published/Produced	Toronto, Ontario: Canadian Scholars' Press, 2016.
Description	494 pages: illustrations; 23 cm
ISBN	9781551308913 (paperback) 9781551308920 (pdf) 9781551308937 (epub)
LC classification	HV5840.C3 C75 2016
Summary	"Substance Use and Abuse provides both students and practitioners in the field of addiction counselling with a foundational working knowledge of psychoactive drugs. It helps the reader understand the bio-psycho-social components of addiction by providing a comprehensive overview of the fundamental concepts and theories of addiction, the major types of psychoactive substances, treatment options and resources, and numerous prevention strategies. It also contains a chapter on the legal, ethical, and practice requirements for becoming a competent addiction counsellor. This new edition has been thoroughly updated to reflect the current issues, theories, and terminology in the addictions field and contains new information on the social dimension of addiction; neurobiology, attachment, and

	environmental stress theories; fetal spectrum disorder and solvent abuse syndrome; drug treatment courts; various new drugs including betel and synthetic cannabis; and new treatment options including internet counselling, narrative therapy, and e-cigarettes."-- Provided by publisher.
LC Subjects	Substance abuse--Canada.
	Substance abuse--Treatment--Canada.
	Drug abuse--Canada.
	Drug abuse--Treatment--Canada.
	Psychotropic drugs.
	Drug addiction.
Notes	Includes bibliographical references and index.
Additional formats	Issued also in electronic format.

Substance use disorders: a guide for the primary care provider

LCCN	2019751983
Type of material	Book
Personal name	Milhorn, H. Thomas, author.
Main title	Substance Use Disorders: A Guide for the Primary Care Provider / by H. Thomas Milhorn.
Edition	1st ed. 2018.
Published/Produced	Cham: Springer International Publishing: Imprint: Springer, 2018.
Description	1 online resource (XXIII, 354 pages 33 illustrations, 31 illustrations in color.)
	PDF
ISBN	9783319630403
Summary	This practical and timely book provides comprehensive, state-of-the-art guidance on how primary care clinicians can best care for patients with substance use disorders. The book covers the major drugs of abuse, as well as the more recent ones, detailing the biology of various addictions and all dimensions of clinical diagnosis and management. It is organized in four parts: (1) The Basics, (2) Psychoactive Substance Dependencies, (3) Diagnosis, Treatment, Recovery, Relapse, and the Family, and (4) Special Groups. Part I, The Basics,

consists of an overview, the various definitions of substance dependence, and the pharmacology of addictive substances. Chapter 1, Overview, is an introductory chapter that covers material common to the entire field of substance dependence. Chapter 2 covers the various definitions of substance dependence, and Chapter 3 reviews the pharmacology of addictive substances. Part II, Psychoactive Substance Dependencies, explains the various drug dependencies-alcohol dependence, sedative-hypnotic dependence, opioid dependence, stimulant dependence, nicotine dependence, cannabis dependence, dissociative dependence, inhalant dependence, hallucinogen dependence, and anabolic steroid dependence. Part III addresses diagnosis, treatment, recovery, relapse, and the family. Part IV, Special Groups, discusses substance dependence in women, adolescents, the elderly, ethnic minority groups, co-occurring disorders, LGBT patients, HIV positive patients, and the impaired physician. In addition to primary care physicians, Substance Use Disorders: A Guide for the Primary Care Provider will serve as an invaluable resource to primary care nurse practitioners and physician assistants, as well as medical students, primary care residents, emergency medicine physicians, ASAM and APA certified addictionists and those studying for certification in those specialties, psychiatrists, psychologists, and alcohol/drug counselors.

Contents   Part I. The Basics - Chapter 1. Overview - Chapter 2. Definitions of Substance Dependence - Chapter 3. Pharmacology of Psychoactive Substances - Part II. Psychoactive Substance Dependencies - Chapter 4. Alcohol Dependence - Chapter 5. Sedative-hypnotic Dependence - Chapter 6. Opioid Dependence - Chapter 7. Stimulant Dependence - Chapter 8. Nicotine Dependence - Chapter 9. Cannabis Dependence - Chapter 10. Dissociative Drug Dependence - Chapter 11. Inhalant Dependence -

	Chapter 12. Hallucinogen Dependence - Chapter 13. Anabolic Steroid Dependence - Part III: Diagnosis, Treatment, Recovery, Relapse, and the Family - Chapter 14. Diagnosis - Chapter 15. Treatment - Chapter 16. Recovery - Chapter 17. Relapse - Chapter 18. The Family - Part IV. Special Groups - Chapter 19. Women - Chapter 20. Adolescents - Chapter 21. The Elderly - Chapter 22. Other Groups - Chapter 23. The Impaired Physician.
LC Subjects	Emergency medicine. General practice (Medicine). Psychiatry.
Other Subjects	General Practice / Family Medicine. Emergency Medicine. Psychiatry.
Additional formats	Print version: Substance use disorders: a guide for the primary care provider 9783319630397 (DLC) 2017947158 Printed edition: 9783319630397 Printed edition: 9783319630410

Synthetic cathinones: novel addictive and stimulatory psychoactive substances

LCCN	2019744784
Type of material	Book
Main title	Synthetic Cathinones: Novel Addictive and Stimulatory Psychoactive Substances / edited by Jolanta B. Zawilska.
Edition	1st ed. 2018.
Published/Produced	Cham: Springer International Publishing: Imprint: Springer, 2018.
Description	1 online resource (X, 207 pages) PDF
ISBN	9783319787077
Related names	Zawilska, Jolanta B. editor.
Summary	Over the last decade a rapidly increasing number of novel psychoactive substance (NPSs), often marketed as "designer drugs", "legal highs", "herbal highs", "research or intermediate chemicals" and "laboratory

	reagents", has appeared on the drug market worldwide in an effort to bypass controlled substance legislation. NPSs encompass a wide range of different compounds and drug classes but had been dominated by synthetic cannabinomimetics and psychostimulatory synthetic cathinones, so-called b-keto amphetamines. Compounds from the later class were first detected in Europe in 2004, and since that time more than 130 new cathinones have been identified and reported to the European Monitoring Centre for Drugs and Drug Addiction. The rapid and extensive worldwide rise of synthetic cathinone abuse is attracting increasing attention, due to many intoxications and overdose deaths.
Contents	Introduction - Novel Psychoactive Substances: classification and General Information - Khat - A Natural Precursor of Synthetic Cathinones - Analytical Techniques for the Detection of Synthetic Cathinones and Their Metabolites - Metabolism of Synthetic Cathinones - Monoamine Transporter and Receptor Interaction Profiles of Synthetic Cathinones - Effects of Synthetic Cathinones on Brain Neurotransmitters - Behavioral Profiles and Underlying Transmitters Circuits of Cathinone-Derived Psychostimulant Drugs of Abuse - Synthetic Cathinones - Prevalence and Motivation of Use - The Effects and Risks Associated with Synthetic Cathinones Use in Humans - Concluding Remarks.
LC Subjects	Neurosciences. Pharmacology.
Other Subjects	Neurosciences. Pharmacology/Toxicology.
Additional formats	Print version: Synthetic cathinones. 9783319787060 (DLC) 2018936185 Printed edition: 9783030087692 Printed edition: 9783319787060 Printed edition: 9783319787084
Series	Current Topics in Neurotoxicity, 2363-9563; 12 Current Topics in Neurotoxicity, 2363-9563; 12

The anthropology of drugs

LCCN	2022060510
Type of material	Book
Personal name	Carrier, Neil C. M., author.
Main title	The anthropology of drugs / Neil Carrier and Lisa L. Gezon.
Published/Produced	New York, NY: Routledge, 2023.
ISBN	9780367625245 (hardback)
	9780367625269 (paperback)
	(ebook)
Related names	Gezon, Lisa L., author.
Summary	"From khat to kava to ketamine, drugs are constitutive parts of cultures, identities, economies and livelihoods. This much-needed book is a clear introduction to the anthropology of drugs, providing a cutting-edge and accessible overview of the topic. The authors examine and assess the following key topics: - How drugs feature in anthropology and the work of anthropologists and the general role of drugs in society - Comparison between biochemical and pharmacological approaches to drugs and bio-socio-cultural models of understanding drugs - Evolutionary origins of psychotropic drug sensitivity and archaeological evidence for the spread of psychoactive substances in pre-history - drugs in spiritual and religions contexts, considering their role in altered states of consciousness, divination, and healing - stimulant drugs and the ambivalence with which they are treated in society - Addiction and dependency - Drug economies, livelihoods and the production and distribution segments of drug commodity chains - Drug policies and drug wars - Drugs, race and gender - The future of the study of drugs and anthropological professional engagements with solving drug problems With the inclusion of chapter summaries and many examples, further reading and case studies-- including drug tourism, drug industries in the Philippines and Mexico, Afghanistan and the 'Golden Triangle' and the opioid

Bibliography

crisis in North America - The Anthropology of Drugs: An Introduction is an ideal introduction for those coming to the topic for the first time, and also for those working in the professional and health sectors. As well as students of anthropology it will be of interest to those in related disciplines including sociology, Psychology, health studies and religion"-- Provided by publisher.

Notes	Includes bibliographical references and index.
Additional formats	Online version: Carrier, Neil C. M. Anthropology of drugs New York, NY: Routledge, 2023 9781003109549 (DLC) 2022060511

The nature of drugs: history, pharmacology, and social impact

LCCN	2021009821
Type of material	Book
Personal name	Shulgin, Alexander T. (Alexander Theodore) author.
Main title	The nature of drugs: history, pharmacology, and social impact / Alexander Shulgin.
Published/Produced	Berkeley: Transform Press, 2021.
Description	1 online resource
ISBN	9780999547229 (ebook)
	(hardback)
LC classification	RM301
Summary	"The Nature of Drugs: History, Pharmacology, and Social Impact, Volume I, was transcribed from the original lecture tapes recorded at SFSU in 1987. Ostensibly taught as an introductory course on drugs and biochemistry, this transcription is a unique document being both a historical record of Sasha's teaching style and the culmination in many ways of his philosophy on drugs, psychopharmacology, states of consciousness, and societal and individual freedoms pertaining to their use, both medicinal and exploratory. The Nature of Drugs is the story of humanity's relationship with psychoactive substances from the perspective of a master psychopharmacologist and will enthrall anyone intrigued by this subject. The Nature of Drugs Presentation The course

168   Bibliography

	will be published in two volumes. Volume I presents Shulgin's view on the origin of drugs, the history of U.S. drug law enforcement, human anatomy, the nervous system, the range of drug administrations, varieties of drug actions, memory and states of consciousness, and research methods. The discussions in Volume I lay the groundwork for Sasha's philosophy on psychopharmacology and society, what defines a drug, the nature of a person's relationship with a given compound, and for extensive examinations of dozens of compounds in Volume II"-- Provided by publisher.
LC Subjects	Drugs--History. Pharmacology--History. Drugs--Research--History. Drugs--Social aspects.
Notes	Includes bibliographical references and index.
Additional formats	Print version: Shulgin, Alexander T. (Alexander Theodore) The nature of drugs Berkeley: Transform Press, 2021. 9780999547212 (DLC) 2021009820

The nature of drugs: history, pharmacology, and social impact

LCCN	2021009820
Type of material	Book
Personal name	Shulgin, Alexander T. (Alexander Theodore) author.
Main title	The nature of drugs: history, pharmacology, and social impact / Alexander Shulgin.
Published/Produced	Berkeley: Transform Press, 2021.
ISBN	9780999547212 (hardback) (ebook)
LC classification	RM301.S518 2021
Summary	"The Nature of Drugs: History, Pharmacology, and Social Impact, Volume I, was transcribed from the original lecture tapes recorded at SFSU in 1987. Ostensibly taught as an introductory course on drugs and biochemistry, this transcription is a unique document being both a historical record of Sasha's teaching style and the culmination in many ways of his philosophy on drugs, psychopharmacology, states

of consciousness, and societal and individual freedoms pertaining to their use, both medicinal and exploratory. The Nature of Drugs is the story of humanity's relationship with psychoactive substances from the perspective of a master psychopharmacologist and will enthrall anyone intrigued by this subject. The Nature of Drugs Presentation The course will be published in two volumes. Volume I presents Shulgin's view on the origin of drugs, the history of U.S. drug law enforcement, human anatomy, the nervous system, the range of drug administrations, varieties of drug actions, memory and states of consciousness, and rescarch methods. The discussions in Volume I lay the groundwork for Sasha's philosophy on psychopharmacology and society, what defines a drug, the nature of a person's relationship with a given compound, and for extensive examinations of dozens of compounds in Volume II"-- Provided by publisher.

LC Subjects	Drugs--History.
	Pharmacology--History.
	Drugs--Research--History.
	Drugs--Social aspects.
Notes	Includes bibliographical references and index.
Additional formats	Online version: Shulgin, Alexander, 1925- The nature of drugs Berkeley: Transform Press, 2021. 9780999547229 (DLC) 2021009821

The pharmakon: concept figure, image of transgression, poetic practice

LCCN	2018394696
Type of material	Book
Main title	The pharmakon: concept figure, image of transgression, poetic practice / edited by Hermann Herlinghaus.
Published/Produced	Heidelberg: Universitätsverlag Winter, [2018]
Description	viii, 392 pages; 21 cm.
ISBN	9783825367404
	3825367401
LC classification	GT3010 .P43 2018

Related names	Herlinghaus, Hermann, 1954- editor.
Summary	The ancient Greek semantic of "pharmakon" comprised at least three meanings-- denoting a medicine, a poison, and/or a magic potion. This helps to uncover a non-dogmatic meaning of "drugs." A millenarian cultural history testifies to the ongoing need of communities and societies to actively use and deal with "pharmaka," prominently including mind-altering substances. However, Western modernity has complicated an unbiased approach to the pharmacological aspects of historical and social life by aggressively multiplying, and later restricting psychoactive substances. The present volume questions a logic of good vs. bad drugs as it discusses a wide semantic spectrum-- the cultural, anthropological, aesthetic, and poetological scope of the "pharmakon." In order to critically resituate the concept, the book offers a glance into compelling scenarios, European, North American, Latin American, Transatlantic, and fascinating transdisciplinary perspectives.
LC Subjects	Drugs--Social aspects.
	Drugs and mass media.
	Drugs and literature.
Notes	Includes bibliographical references and index.
Series	Beiträge zur Philosophie. Neue Folge
	Beiträge zur Philosophie. Neue Folge.

The Routledge companion to ecstatic experience in the ancient world

LCCN	2021018966
Type of material	Book
Main title	The Routledge companion to ecstatic experience in the ancient world / edited by Diana L. Stein, Sarah Kielt Costello, and Karen Polinger Foster.
Published/Produced	Abingdon, Oxon; New York, NY: Routledge, 2022.
Description	1 online resource
ISBN	9781000464764 (epub)
	9781003041610 (ebook)
	(hardback)

	(paperback)
LC classification	GN472.4
Portion of title	Companion to ecstatic experience in the ancient world
Related names	Stein, Diana L., editor.
	Costello, Sarah Kielt, 1971- editor.
	Foster, Karen Polinger, 1950- editor.
Summary	"For millennia, people have universally engaged in ecstatic experience as an essential element in ritual practice, spiritual belief and cultural identification. This volume offers the first systematic investigation of its myriad roles and manifestations in the ancient Mediterranean and Near East. The twenty-nine contributors represent a broad range of scholarly disciplines, seeking answers to fundamental questions regarding the patterns and commonalities of this vital aspect of the past. How was the experience construed and by what means was it achieved? Who was involved? Where and when were its rites carried out? How was it reflected in pictorial arts and written records? What was its relation to other components of the sociocultural compact? In proposing responses, the authors draw upon a wealth of original research in many fields, generating new perspectives and thought-provoking, often surprising, conclusions. With their abundant cross-cultural and cross-temporal references, the chapters mutually enrich each other and collectively deepen our understanding of ecstatic phenomena thousands of years ago. Another noteworthy feature of the book is its illustrative content, including commissioned reconstructions of ecstatic scenarios and pairings of works of Bronze Age and modern psychedelic art. Scholars, students and other readers interested in antiquity, comparative religion and the social and cognitive sciences will find much to explore in the fascinating realm of ecstatic experience in the ancient world"-- Provided by publisher.

Contents

Introduction / Diana L. Stein, Sarah Kielt Costello and Karen Polinger Foster - Contextualizing the study of ecstatic experience in ancient old world societies / Sarah Kielt Costello - Not only ecstasy: pouring new concepts into old vessels / Etzel Cardeña - From shamans to sorcerers: empirical models for defining ritual practices and ecstatic experience in ancient, medieval and modern societies / Michael J. Winkelman - Psychoactive plants in the ancient world: observations of an ethnobotanist / Giorgio Samorini - Ecstasy meets paleoethnobotany: botanical stimulants in ancient Inner Asia / Alison Betts - Caucasian cocktails: the early use of alcohol in 'the cradle of wine' / Stephen Batiuk - Mind-altering plants in Babylonian medical sources / Barbara Böck - Plant-based potions and ecstatic states in Hittite rituals / Rita Francia - Forbidden at Philae: proscription of aphrodisiac and psychoactive plants in Ptolemaic Egypt / Riccardo Andreozzi and Claudia Sarkady - The Ring-Kernos and psychotropic substances / David Ilan - Beer, beasts and bodies: shedding boundaries in bounded spaces / Anne Porter - Lament, spectacle and emotion in a ritual for Ishtar / Sam Mirelman - Writing for the dead, welcoming the solar-eye goddess and ecstatic expression in Egyptian religion / John Coleman Darnell - Altered states on prepalatial Crete / Emily Miller Bonney - Bodies in ecstasy: shamanic elements in Minoan religion / Christine Morris and Alan Peatfield - The Mycenaeans and ecstatic ritual experience / Susan Lupack - Emotional arousal, sensory deprivation and 'miraculous healing' in the cult of Asclepius / Olympia Panagiotidou - Ecstasy and initiation in the Eleusinian mysteries / Alice Clinch - Apolline and Dionysian ecstasy at Delphi / Yulia Ustinova - Communing with the spirits: funeral processions in ancient Rome / Maik Patzelt - Ecstatic experience and possession disorders in ancient Mesopotamia / Ulrike Steinert - Ghosts in and outside the machine: a

	phenomenology of intelligence, psychic possession and prophetic ecstasy in ancient Mesopotamia / John Z. Wee - Ecstatic speech in ancient Mesopotamia / Benjamin R. Foster - Ecstatic experience: the prototheme of a Near Eastern glyptic language family / Diana L. Stein - Understanding the language of trees: ecstatic experience and interspecies communication in late Bronze Age Crete / Caroline J. Tully - Psychedelic art and ecstatic visions in the Aegean / Karen Polinger Foster - Sight as ecstatic experience in the ancient Mediterranean / Nassos Papalexandrou.
LC Subjects	Ecstasy--Mediterranean Region--History--To 1500. Hallucinogenic drugs and religious experience--Mediterranean Region--History--To 1500. Bronze age--Mediterranean Region. Mediterranean Region--Religious life and customs--History--To 1500.
Notes	Includes bibliographical references and index.
Additional formats	Print version: Routledge companion to ecstatic experience in the ancient world Abingdon, Oxon; New York, NY: Routledge, 2022 9780367480325 (DLC) 2021018965

The Routledge companion to ecstatic experience in the ancient world

LCCN	2021018965
Type of material	Book
Main title	The Routledge companion to ecstatic experience in the ancient world / edited by Diana L. Stein, Sarah Kielt Costello, and Karen Polinger Foster.
Published/Produced	Abingdon, Oxon; New York, NY: Routledge, 2022.
ISBN	9780367480325 (hardback)
	9781032108483 (paperback)
	(ebook)
LC classification	GN472.4.R68 2022
Portion of title	Companion to ecstatic experience in the ancient world
Related names	Stein, Diana L., editor.
	Costello, Sarah Kielt, 1971- editor.
	Foster, Karen Polinger, 1950- editor.

Summary

"For millennia, people have universally engaged in ecstatic experience as an essential element in ritual practice, spiritual belief and cultural identification. This volume offers the first systematic investigation of its myriad roles and manifestations in the ancient Mediterranean and Near East. The twenty-nine contributors represent a broad range of scholarly disciplines, seeking answers to fundamental questions regarding the patterns and commonalities of this vital aspect of the past. How was the experience construed and by what means was it achieved? Who was involved? Where and when were its rites carried out? How was it reflected in pictorial arts and written records? What was its relation to other components of the sociocultural compact? In proposing responses, the authors draw upon a wealth of original research in many fields, generating new perspectives and thought-provoking, often surprising, conclusions. With their abundant cross-cultural and cross-temporal references, the chapters mutually enrich each other and collectively deepen our understanding of ecstatic phenomena thousands of years ago. Another noteworthy feature of the book is its illustrative content, including commissioned reconstructions of ecstatic scenarios and pairings of works of Bronze Age and modern psychedelic art. Scholars, students and other readers interested in antiquity, comparative religion and the social and cognitive sciences will find much to explore in the fascinating realm of ecstatic experience in the ancient world"-- Provided by publisher.

Contents

Introduction / Diana L. Stein, Sarah Kielt Costello and Karen Polinger Foster - Contextualizing the study of ecstatic experience in ancient old world societies / Sarah Kielt Costello - Not only ecstasy: pouring new concepts into old vessels / Etzel Cardeña - From shamans to sorcerers: empirical models for defining ritual practices and ecstatic experience in ancient, medieval and modern societies / Michael J.

Winkelman - Psychoactive plants in the ancient world: observations of an ethnobotanist / Giorgio Samorini - Ecstasy meets paleoethnobotany: botanical stimulants in ancient Inner Asia / Alison Betts - Caucasian cocktails: the early use of alcohol in 'the cradle of wine' / Stephen Batiuk - Mind-altering plants in Babylonian medical sources / Barbara Böck - Plant-based potions and ecstatic states in Hittite rituals / Rita Francia - Forbidden at Philae: proscription of aphrodisiac and psychoactive plants in Ptolemaic Egypt / Riccardo Andreozzi and Claudia Sarkady - The Ring-Kernos and psychotropic substances / David Ilan - Beer, beasts and bodies: shedding boundaries in bounded spaces / Anne Porter - Lament, spectacle and emotion in a ritual for Ishtar / Sam Mirelman - Writing for the dead, welcoming the solar-eye goddess and ecstatic expression in Egyptian religion / John Coleman Darnell - Altered states on prepalatial Crete / Emily Miller Bonney - Bodies in ecstasy: shamanic elements in Minoan religion / Christine Morris and Alan Peatfield - The Mycenaeans and ecstatic ritual experience / Susan Lupack - Emotional arousal, sensory deprivation and 'miraculous healing' in the cult of Asclepius / Olympia Panagiotidou - Ecstasy and initiation in the Eleusinian mysteries / Alice Clinch - Apolline and Dionysian ecstasy at Delphi / Yulia Ustinova - Communing with the spirits: funeral processions in ancient Rome / Maik Patzelt - Ecstatic experience and possession disorders in ancient Mesopotamia / Ulrike Steinert - Ghosts in and outside the machine: a phenomenology of intelligence, psychic possession and prophetic ecstasy in ancient Mesopotamia / John Z. Wee - Ecstatic speech in ancient Mesopotamia / Benjamin R. Foster - Ecstatic experience: the proto-theme of a Near Eastern glyptic language family / Diana L. Stein - Understanding the language of trees: ecstatic experience and interspecies communication in late Bronze Age Crete / Caroline J. Tully -

LC Subjects	Psychedelic art and ecstatic visions in the Aegean / Karen Polinger Foster - Sight as ecstatic experience in the ancient Mediterranean / Nassos Papalexandrou. Ecstasy--Mediterranean Region--History--To 1500. Hallucinogenic drugs and religious experience--Mediterranean Region--History--To 1500. Bronze age--Mediterranean Region. Mediterranean Region--Religious life and customs--History--To 1500.
Notes	Includes bibliographical references and index.
Additional formats	Online version: Routledge companion to ecstatic experience in the ancient world Abingdon, Oxon; New York, NY: Routledge, 2022 9781003041610 (DLC) 2021018966

The social cost of legal and illegal drugs in Belgium

LCCN	2016519747
Type of material	Book
Personal name	Lievens, Delfine, author.
Main title	The social cost of legal and illegal drugs in Belgium / Delfine Lievens .... [and 7 others].
Published/Produced	Antwerpen: Maklu, 2016.
Description	422 pages: illustrations; 23 cm
ISBN	9789046608166
	9046608166
LC classification	HV5840.B42 L55 2016
Related names	Rijksuniversiteit te Gent. Institute for International Research on Criminal Policy, issuing body.
Summary	Alcohol, tobacco, illegal drugs and psychoactive medication (mis)use are associated with a higher likelihood of developing several diseases, (traffic) injuries and crimes. These substances reduce quality of life and increase the health care and law enforcement costs, productivity losses, etc. Consequently, the social and economic impact of substances on society is substantial. The SOCOST study estimates for the first time social costs for alcohol, tobacco, illegal drugs and psychoactive medication in Belgium for the year 2012. This cost-

Bibliography

	of-illness study presents the direct costs, the indirect cost as well as the intangible costs related to substance (mis)use. This research was commissioned by the Belgian Federal Science Policy Office (BELSPO) in the framework of the Federal Research Programme Drugs. Two universities cooperated: Ghent University, Institute for International Research on Criminal Policy (IRCP) and the Vrije Universiteit Brussel, Interuniversity Centre for Health Economics Research (I-CHER).
LC Subjects	Drug abuse--Economic aspects--Belgium.
	Drug abuse--Social aspects--Belgium.
	Drug abuse--Health aspects--Belgium.
	Drug abuse--Law and legislation--Belgium.
Notes	Includes bibliographical references.
Series	IRCP research series; volume 51
	IRCP-series; v. 51.

Using substances to enhance performance: a psychology of neuroenhancement

LCCN	2020405263
Type of material	Book
Main title	Using substances to enhance performance: a Psychology of neuroenhancement / topic editors, Wanja Wolff, University of Konstanz, Germany, Ralf Brand, University of Potsdam, Germany.
Published/Produced	[Lausanne, Switzerland]: Frontiers Media SA [2017]
Description	1 online resource (114 pages)
Rights advisory	Creative Commons Attribution 4.0 International. CC BY 4.0 https://creativecommons.org/licenses/by/4.0/
Access advisory	Unrestricted online access
Links	https://hdl.loc.gov/loc.gdc/gdcebookspublic.2020405263
ISBN	9782889450756
LC classification	QP376
Related names	Brand, Ralf, editor.
	Wolff, Wanja, editor.
Summary	"Neuroenhancement (NE) is a behavior conceptualized as the use of a potentially

psychoactive substance to enhance ones' already proficient cognitive capacities. Depending on the specific definitions used, prevalence estimates vary greatly between very low 0.3% (for illicit substances) to astonishingly high 89% (for freely available lifestyle substances). These variations indicate that further research and more conceptual and theoretical clarification of the NE construct is dearly needed. The contributions of this research topic aim to do just that. Specific questions addressed are: How prevalent is NE behavior? How can NE research profit from the already more evolved field of social science research on doping in sports? How is NE perceived by the public? What psychological processes and variables play a role in the decision to neuroenhance? A wide array of methodological approaches is used to investigate these questions. The topics contributions range from theoretical to experimental accounts on NE, and they utilize a diverse set of methods ranging from qualitative to neuroscientific approaches. The research presented here represents a first step towards what we have labeled a psychological approach to NE. By addressing the questions above, this research topic hopefully advances our understanding of NE behavior. As with every new field of research, new answers always prompt new questions. In light of what we know now about NE, we hope that the findings presented here will be pursued by other researchers in the future. Clearly, the endeavor to understand NE behavior has only just begun."--Page 2.

LC Subjects	Brain chemistry.
	Central nervous system stimulants.
Notes	"Published in: Frontiers in Psychology."
	Includes bibliographical references.
Series	Frontiers Research Topics

Index

A

analysis, 6, 11, 13, 14, 15, 16, 18, 19, 21, 24, 26, 27, 29, 31, 39, 40, 41, 45, 46, 47, 48, 49, 50, 51, 52, 56, 57, 62, 63, 64, 65, 68, 69, 71, 73, 74, 77, 78, 89, 90, 91, 92, 95, 97, 105, 118, 125, 126, 127, 128, 129, 130, 149, 151, 152, 158, 160
anthropogenic marker, v, vii, viii, 23, 24, 25, 38, 41

B

benchmarking, 37
benzodiazepine, v, vii, ix, 59, 60, 61, 75

C

caffeine, v, vii, viii, 19, 23, 24, 25, 26, 27, 28, 29, 30, 31, 32, 34, 36, 37, 38, 40, 41, 84, 86, 101, 137
chemical(s), vii, 2, 3, 4, 5, 6, 9, 10, 12, 13, 14, 15, 19, 24, 25, 26, 40, 41, 61, 62, 63, 64, 73, 81, 83, 95, 97, 98, 111, 112, 115, 124, 128, 129, 134, 145, 160, 164
chromatographic, v, vii, 27, 43, 47, 64, 71, 95, 96
chromatography, ix, 17, 26, 59, 62, 75, 106, 127, 128, 129, 130
clinical, ix, 6, 7, 41, 45, 52, 57, 59, 61, 62, 68, 69, 71, 72, 73, 75, 85, 99, 100, 103, 104, 105, 121, 122, 127, 128, 129, 130, 132, 148, 149, 152, 162
concentration(s), viii, 6, 12, 19, 24, 28, 29, 30, 31, 32, 36, 37, 39, 43, 45, 46, 47, 48, 49, 51, 52, 53, 54, 55, 63, 64, 65, 66, 67, 68, 69, 70, 71, 74, 85
correlation(s), viii, 20, 23, 26, 29, 31, 49, 51, 65, 66, 71
CYP2D6, v, vii, viii, 43, 44, 45, 46, 47, 49, 50, 51, 52, 53, 54, 55, 56, 57

D

detection, viii, ix, 7, 15, 23, 26, 39, 41, 47, 59, 62, 64, 66, 68, 71, 72, 74, 76, 77, 91, 107, 126, 127, 151, 165
development, v, vii, 7, 16, 19, 55, 56, 59, 63, 65, 75, 76, 77, 84, 86, 88, 89, 93, 122, 147
diagnosis, 45, 57, 73, 93, 100, 127, 129, 135, 162, 164
drug(s), vii, viii, ix, 1, 3, 4, 5, 7, 8, 9, 10, 11, 12, 13, 15, 16, 17, 19, 24, 25, 39, 40, 41, 42, 43, 44, 45, 46, 49, 51, 52, 53, 54, 55, 56, 57, 59, 60, 61, 62, 71, 72, 73, 74, 75, 76, 77, 78, 79, 84, 86, 97, 101, 103, 104, 105, 106, 107, 108, 109, 110, 111, 112, 114, 115, 117, 118, 120, 121, 123, 124, 125, 126, 127, 129, 131, 132, 133, 135, 136, 137, 138, 140, 143, 144, 145, 149, 150, 151, 152, 153, 154, 155, 157, 159, 160, 161, 162, 163, 164, 165, 166, 167, 168, 169, 170, 173, 176, 177

E

economy, vii, 1
efficiency, viii, 2, 29, 30, 37, 45, 54
element(s), vii, 1, 20, 21, 171, 172, 174, 175

equipment, 26, 29, 62
expression(s), v, vii, 3, 43, 46, 47, 49, 50, 52, 53, 54, 55, 85, 172, 175
extraction, 26, 28, 30, 37, 38, 49, 64, 69, 71, 91, 95, 96

F

forensic(s), ix, 1, 6, 16, 17, 18, 19, 20, 23, 40, 43, 52, 56, 57, 59, 61, 62, 68, 69, 71, 72, 73, 74, 75, 76, 102, 105, 125, 127, 128, 129, 142, 148, 149, 150
formulation(s), vii, 2

G

gene, ix, 43, 44, 45, 46, 47, 49, 50, 51, 52, 53, 54, 55, 56, 85
gene copy number, ix, 43, 44, 45, 46, 49, 51, 52, 53, 55
genetic(s), 44, 45, 46, 54, 56, 57, 85, 105

H

hazardous, v, 1, 41, 98, 99, 123
high performance liquid chromatography (HPLC), 60, 62, 63, 64, 65, 66, 67, 68, 69, 71, 72, 76, 77, 79

I

identification, ix, 59, 62, 63, 75, 171, 174
illicit drugs, 2, 14, 18, 19, 21, 39, 40, 84
inadequate, ix, 59
innovative, viii, 2
instrumentation, 27, 63

L

legal highs, vii, 1, 2, 4, 60, 139, 140, 151, 152, 164
liquid chromatography-tandem mass spectrometry (LC-MS/MS), v, viii, 23, 24, 26, 27, 29, 38, 46, 47, 49, 52, 55, 62, 71
liquid(s), viii, ix, 17, 23, 26, 31, 46, 49, 59, 62, 98, 106

M

manufacturing, vii, 2, 3
measurement(s), 30, 32, 36, 39, 55, 67, 76
metabolite ratio, 44
method validation, viii, 24, 30, 31, 32, 37, 39, 41, 72

N

new psychoactive substances (NPS), v, vii, ix, 1, 2, 3, 4, 5, 7, 8, 10, 11, 12, 13, 14, 15, 16, 17, 59, 60, 61, 62, 71, 72, 74, 75, 90, 98, 103, 104, 106, 124, 125, 126, 127, 129, 130, 132, 135, 141, 145, 146, 148, 149, 150, 151, 152
NPS-benzodiazepine, ix, 59, 60, 61, 62, 71, 72

P

parameter(s), viii, 23, 26, 29, 30, 32, 37, 38, 48, 65
patient(s), viii, 20, 43, 44, 45, 46, 49, 50, 51, 52, 53, 54, 55, 56, 75, 82, 83, 86, 100, 102, 107, 122, 162
pattern(s), v, vii, 8, 9, 10, 13, 43, 49, 50, 54, 103, 104, 112, 115, 126, 130, 132, 171, 174
performance(s), ix, 10, 29, 30, 37, 48, 59, 62, 107, 111, 130, 132, 177
pharmacogenetic, v, vii, 43, 45, 56
pharmacology, 6, 9, 56, 57, 73, 75, 120, 121, 122, 123, 125, 132, 133, 146, 148, 149, 150, 151, 163, 165, 167, 168, 169
phenazepam, v, vii, ix, 59, 60, 61, 62, 63, 65, 66, 68, 69, 70, 71, 72, 73, 74, 75
pollutant(s), viii, 23, 25, 26, 95, 97
population(s), ix, 10, 12, 13, 15, 24, 38, 40, 41, 43, 44, 52, 53, 55, 56, 57, 79, 100, 101, 141
preparation, 26, 28, 46, 49, 63, 64, 95, 96, 99
psychiatric patients, viii, 43, 44, 45, 52, 54, 55

Index

psychoactive, vii, ix, 1, 2, 3, 4, 15, 16, 59, 60, 72, 74, 75, 82, 83, 86, 87, 88, 89, 93, 95, 97, 101, 103, 104, 108, 109, 110, 112, 115, 118, 120, 122, 124, 126, 130, 132, 134, 136, 137, 139, 143, 144, 147, 149, 150, 151, 152, 153, 154, 155, 156, 157, 158, 159,160, 161, 162, 163, 164, 165, 166, 167, 169, 170, 172, 175, 176, 178

R

reappearance, ix, 59
recreational, ix, 4, 6, 8, 9, 59, 69, 71, 73, 124, 126, 131, 133, 139, 151
reverse-phase, ix, 59

S

sample(s), v, vii, viii, ix, 6, 7, 12, 19, 20, 23, 24, 26, 28, 30, 32, 37, 38, 43, 45, 46, 47, 49, 50, 51, 53, 54, 55, 56, 60, 62, 63, 64, 69, 70, 71, 72, 77, 91, 94, 96, 125
severe, ix, 3, 10, 54, 59
solid-phase extraction (SPE), viii, 24, 26, 28
stability, 25, 28, 37, 91
statistical, 30, 31, 37, 49, 51, 53
substance(s), vii, ix, 1, 2, 3, 4, 6, 7, 8, 9, 10, 11, 12, 13, 14, 15, 16, 44, 46, 49, 52, 53, 54, 55, 59, 60, 63, 72, 74, 75, 82, 83, 84, 86, 87, 88, 89, 93, 95, 97, 99, 100, 101, 102, 103, 104, 107, 108, 109, 110, 112, 115, 118, 119, 122, 124, 126, 127, 129, 130, 132, 134, 135, 136, 137, 138, 139, 143, 144, 147, 149, 150, 151, 152, 153, 154, 155, 156, 157, 158, 159, 160, 161, 162, 163, 164, 165, 166, 167, 169, 170, 172, 175, 176, 177, 178

surface water, viii, 24, 25, 37, 38, 42
synthetic cannabinoids, vii, viii, 2, 3, 4, 5, 6, 7, 8, 11, 60, 71, 106, 125, 126, 131, 133, 149, 155, 156
synthetic cathinones, viii, 2, 8, 10, 11, 122, 131, 133, 164, 165

T

therapeutic, ix, 3, 45, 52, 59, 72, 81, 83, 86, 122, 143, 144
toxicology, 6, 9, 16, 17, 18, 40, 56, 72, 73, 74, 75, 95, 97, 99, 106, 107, 125, 127, 128, 129, 146, 148, 149, 150, 151, 165
treatment(s), ix, 4, 6, 11, 15, 19, 21, 25, 37, 39, 42, 44, 45, 52, 53, 54, 55, 56, 57, 59, 60, 64, 75, 76, 77, 81, 82, 83, 85, 86, 87, 88, 89, 100, 101, 111, 114, 117, 131, 133, 140, 155, 157, 161, 162, 164

U

ultraviolet, ix, 59, 62

V

validation, v, vii, viii, ix, 23, 26, 29, 30, 31, 36, 38, 40, 41, 60, 63, 64, 66, 74, 76, 77, 79
variant(s), v, vii, 43, 46, 119, 135
visible, ix, 59, 62

W

warning system, 13, 14, 16
water, v, vii, viii, 6, 15, 19, 21, 23, 25, 26, 27, 28, 30, 31, 34, 35, 37, 38, 39, 41, 42, 46, 63, 64, 66, 76, 78, 95, 97, 126